GETTING WELL NATURALLY SERIES

Stomach Ailments and Digestive Disturbances

Michael T. Murray, N.D.

D1044474

PRIMA PUBLISHING

PRIMA PUBLISHING and its colophon are registered trademarks of Prima Communications, Inc.

Warning—Disclaimer

Prima Publishing has designed this book to provide information in regard to the subject matter covered. It is sold with the understanding that the publisher and the author are not liable for the misconception or misuse of information provided. Every effort has been made to make this book as complete and as accurate as possible. The purpose of this book is to educate. The author and Prima Publishing shall have neither liability nor responsibility to any person or entity with respect to any loss, damage, or injury caused or alleged to be caused directly or indirectly by the information contained in this book. The information presented herein is in no way intended as a substitute for medical counseling.

Library of Congress Cataloging-in-Publication Data

Murray, Michael T.
    Stomach ailments and digestive disturbances : how you can benefit from diet, vitamins, minerals, herbs, exercise, and other natural methods / Michael T. Murray.
        p.   cm.
    Includes bibiliographical references and index.
    ISBN 0-7615-0657-8
        1. Stomach—Diseases—Alternative treatment.   2. Indigestion— Alternative treatment.   3. Naturopathy.   I. Title.
    RC827.M87   1997
    616.3'306—dc21   97-10373
                                                                  CIP

97 98 99 00 01 HH 10 9 8 7 6 5 4 3 2
Printed in the United States of America

All products mentioned in this book are trademarks of their respective companies.

How to Order

Single copies may be ordered from Prima Publishing, P.O. Box 1260, Rocklin, CA 95677; telephone (916) 632-4400. Quantity discounts are also available. On your letterhead, include information concerning the intended use of the books and the number of books you wish to purchase.

Visit us online at http://www.primapublishing.com

Contents

Before You Read On

This book was written to empower you regarding your health care decisions; it is not designed to replace appropriate medical care. With that in mind, here are some important recommendations:

- Do not self-diagnose. Proper medical care is critical to good health. If you have symptoms suggestive of an illness, please consult a physician—preferably a naturopath, holistic physician or osteopath, chiropractor, or other natural health care specialist.

- If you are currently on a prescription medication, you absolutely must consult your doctor before discontinuing it. Furthermore, you must make your physician aware of all the nutritional supplements you are currently taking and why.

- If you wish to try a nutritional supplement as a therapeutic measure, discuss it with your physician. Since he or she is most likely unaware of the natural alternatives available, you may need to do some educating. Bring this book along with you to the doctor's office. The natural alternatives being recommended are based on published studies in medical journals. Key references are provided if your physician wants additional information.

• Remember, although many nutritional alternatives, such as nutritional supplements and planted-based medicines, are effective on their own, they work even better if they are part of a comprehensive natural treatment plan that focuses on diet and lifestyle.

About the Author

Michael T. Murray, N.D., is widely regarded as one of the world's leading authorities on natural medicine. He is a graduate, faculty member, and member of the Board of Trustees of Bastyr University in Seattle, Washington. In addition to maintaining a private medical practice, Dr. Murray is an accomplished writer, educator, and lecturer. He is the medical editor of *The American Journal of Natural Medicine.*

Dr. Murray serves on several editorial boards and advisory panels. As a consultant to the health food industry, Dr. Murray has been instrumental in bringing many effective natural products to America, including: ginkgo biloba extract, glucosamine sulfate, silymarin, enteric-coated peppermint oil, bilberry extract, DGL (deglycyrrhizinated licorice), saw palmetto berry extract, and the first thermogenic formula for weight loss.

1

The Digestive System—
Function and Analysis

In order to gain the benefits from the foods that we eat it is critical that they be properly digested, absorbed, and eliminated. The best nutrition in the world will go to waste if the body is unable to process it. Fortunately, the human digestive system usually is quite efficient in extracting the necessary nutrients from foods.

The major function of the gastrointestinal (digestive) system is to break down and absorb nutrients. The digestive system extends from the mouth to the anus. It consists of the gastrointestinal tract and its appendage organs: the salivary glands, the liver and gallbladder, and the pancreas.

Digestion occurs as a result of both mechanical and chemical processes. The mechanical processes of digestion are brought about by grinding, crushing, and mixing of the food mass with digestive juices during propulsion through the digestive tract. The digestive juices are responsible for the chemical breakdown of food. The active compounds in the digestive juices are primarily enzymes.

Where Does Digestion Begin?

The digestive process begins in the mouth. Chewing food thoroughly is the first step toward getting the most from the food you eat. Chewing signals other components of the digestive system to get ready to go to work; it also allows food to mix with saliva. Saliva contains the enzyme salivary amylase, which breaks down starch molecules into smaller sugars. Once the food has been chewed, it is transported by the esophagus into the stomach.

The Role of the Stomach

Food is broken down in the stomach by mechanical as well as chemical means. The stomach churns and gyrates to promote the mixing of the food with its digestive secretions, including hydrochloric acid and the enzyme pepsin. These factors are critical to proper protein digestion and mineral absorption. If hydrochloric acid secretion is insufficient or inhibited, proper protein digestion will not occur. Food remains in the stomach until it is reduced to a semiliquid consistency. In general, this process takes anywhere from 45 minutes to 4 hours. Once the food material leaves the stomach, it is referred to as chyme.

The Role of the Small Intestine

It takes chyme approximately 2 to 4 hours to make its way through the 21-foot-long small intestine. The small intestine is divided into three segments: The duodenum is the first 10 to 12 inches, the jejunum is the middle portion and about 8 feet long, and the ileum is about 12 feet long. The small intestine participates in all aspects of digestion, absorption, and transport of ingested materials. It secretes a variety of digestive and protective substances as well as receiving the secretions of the pancreas, liver, and gallbladder.

Absorption of minerals occurs predominantly in the duodenum; absorption of water-soluble vitamins, carbohydrates, and protein occurs primarily in the jejunum; and the ileum absorbs fat-soluble vitamins, fat, cholesterol, and bile salts. Diseases involving the small intestine often result in malabsorption syndromes characterized by multiple nutrient deficiencies. Common causes of malabsorption include celiac disease (gluten intolerance), food allergies or intolerances, intestinal infections, and Crohn's disease.

The Role of Pancreatic Enzymes

The pancreas produces enzymes that are required for the digestion and absorption of food. Each day the pancreas secretes about 1.5 quarts of pancreatic juice into the small intestine. Enzymes secreted include lipases, amylases, and proteases.

Lipases, along with bile, function in the digestion of fats. Deficiency of lipase results in malabsorption of fats and fat-soluble vitamins. Amylases break down starch molecules into smaller sugars. (Amylase is secreted by the salivary glands as well as the pancreas.) The proteases secreted by the pancreas (trypsin, chymotrypsin, and carboxypeptidase) function in digestion by breaking down protein molecules into single amino acids. Incomplete digestion of proteins creates a number of problems including the development of allergies and formation of toxic substances produced during putrefaction. Putrefaction refers to the breakdown of protein material by bacteria.

The proteases serve several other important functions. They are largely responsible for keeping the small intestine free from parasites (including bacteria, yeast, protozoa, and intestinal worms).[1] A lack of proteases or other digestive secretions greatly increases an individual's risk of intestinal infections, including chronic candida infections of the gastrointestinal tract. The proteases also are important in preventing tissue damage during inflammation, the formation of fibrin clots, and the depositing of immune complexes in body tissues.[2]

The Role of the Liver and Biliary System

The liver manufactures bile, an extremely important substance in the absorption of fats, oils, and fat-soluble vitamins. Bile produced by the liver is either secreted into the small intestine or stored in the gallbladder. Bile also plays an important role in making the stool soft by promoting the incorporation of water into the stool. Without enough bile, the stool can become quite hard and difficult to pass.

Like pancreatic enzymes, bile also serves to keep the small intestine free from unwanted microorganisms. Each day about 1 quart of bile is secreted into the small intestine. About 99% of what is excreted in the bile (including bile acids and excreted toxins) is reabsorbed back into the body via the gastrointestinal tract.

When additional bile acids are ingested, usually as ox bile, they are known to increase the output of bile and help promote a mild laxative effect. For this reason, many commercial digestive aids contain ox bile. Another method of increasing the output of bile is by using nutritional formulas containing choline and methionine. A daily dose of 1,000 mg of choline and 500 mg of methionine is sufficient in most cases to increase bile flow.

The Role of the Large Intestine (Colon)

The large intestine is about 5 feet long and functions in the absorption of water, electrolytes (salts), and, in limited amounts, some of the final products of digestion. The large intestine also provides temporary storage for waste products. The health of the colon is largely determined by the types of foods that are eaten. In particular, dietary fiber is of critical importance in maintaining the health of the colon. Equally as important as proper digestion is the proper elimination of waste products. A bowel movement every 12 to 24 hours is critical to good health. This proper elimination requires a diet high in dietary fiber. Such a diet is rich in fruits, vegetables, whole grains, legumes, nuts, and seeds. A high-fiber diet increases both the frequency and quantity of bowel movements, decreases the transit time of stools, decreases the absorption of toxins from the stool, and appears to be a preventive factor in several diseases that affect the colon, including constipation, colon cancer, diverticulitis (inflammation or infection of small outpouchings of the intestines), hemorrhoids, and the irritable bowel syndrome. Several of these conditions (with the exception of colon cancer) are discussed more fully in Chapter 5.

The Need for Proper Evaluation

The digestive system is a truly integrated system: The function of one aspect usually affects the others. This interrelationship among the components of the digestive system often makes determining the exact cause of a digestive disturbance difficult. Evaluating digestive symptoms/disturbances without the aid of a physician can be very frustrating and yet proper evaluation is absolutely essential to developing effective treatment. To find a physician in your area who may be familiar with the recommendations contained in this book, contact the following organizations:

The American Association of Naturopathic Physicians
P.O. Box 20386
Seattle, WA 98102
(206) 323-7610

The American Holistic Medical Association
4101 Lake Boone Trail, #201
Raleigh, NC 26707
(919) 787-5146

American College of Advancement in Medicine (ACAM)
23121 Verdugo Drive, Suite 204
Laguna Hills, CA 92653
1-800-532-3688 (outside California)
   or 1-800-435-6199 (inside California)

Comprehensive Digestive Stool Analysis

One of the most useful tools in determining the possible causes of digestive disturbance is the comprehensive digestive stool analysis—a battery of integrated diagnostic laboratory tests that evaluate digestion, intestinal function, intestinal environment, and absorption by carefully examining the stool.[3] Laboratories that I am familiar with that provide this often necessary battery of tests are:

Great Smokies Diagnostic Laboratory (1-800-522-4762)
National BioTech Laboratory (1-800-846-6285)
Diagnos-Techs (1-800-87-TESTS)
Meridian Valley Clinical Laboratory (1-206-859-8700)

All of these laboratories are quite good. For simplicity, I will refer to the comprehensive digestive stool analysis performed by these labs as CDSA.

The CDSA performed by these laboratories provides information that is useful in leading to the correct diagnosis of causes and the development of appropriate therapeutic resources. Many physicians consider it a "foundation" screening test that consistently provides valuable clinical information. The CDSA can uncover the causes of both acute and chronic illnesses. The test involves following a special diet for at least two days. Each lab has slightly different recommendations: Basically the goal is to eat a variety of foods and avoid laxatives, iron supplements, vitamin C, multivitamin formulas, and digestive enzymes as they may interfere with test results.

Since I have the most experience with Great Smokies Diagnostic Laboratory and their CDSA, I will use this test as an example of what a complete evaluation should include in the discussion below of individual components of CSDA.* The other laboratories mentioned offer similar versions to Great Smokies' CDSA. Here are the individual components that should be analyzed, followed by a brief discussion of their significance:

Digestion

 Triglycerides

 Chymotrypsin

 Meat fibers

 Vegetable fibers

 Valerate, iso-Butyrate

Absorption

 Long-chain fatty acids

 Cholesterol

 Total fecal fat

 Total short-chain fatty acids

---

*Much of the information provided here is derived from a chapter on "Comprehensive Digestive Stool Analysis" in *A Textbook of Natural Medicine* (Bastyr University Publications, 1995) by Stephen Barrie, N.D., as well as well-referenced education materials prepared by Great Smokies Diagnostic Laboratory.

Colonic Environment
    Beneficial bacteria
        Lactobacillus
        Bifidobacteria
        E. Coli
    Pathogenic bacteria
    Mycology
    Metabolic Markers
        pH
        Short-chain fatty acid distribution
        Butyrate
        Beta-Glucuronidase
    Immunology
        Fecal secretory IgA
    Dysbiosis index
    Macroscopic
        Fecal color
        Mucus
        Occult blood

Digestion

Triglycerides [Reference range: <0.3%] Triglycerides are the major dietary fat component. Elevated levels of triglycerides in the stool reflect incomplete fat breakdown by pancreatic lipase and suggest pancreatic insufficiency.

Chymotrypsin [Reference range: 6.2 to 41.0 IU/g] Fecal chymotrypsin is a measure of proteolytic enzyme activity that is both sensitive and specific. Chymotrypsin activity in the stool is closely correlated with activity in the duodenum and small intestine. Decreased quantitative fecal values reflect pancreatic insufficiency or decreased hydrochloric acid output by the stomach. As a consequence, there is potential incomplete digestion of proteins, food allergies, bacterial and candida overgrowth in the small intestine, and an increased risk for parasitic infections. Elevated levels of chymotrypsin suggest that food is traveling too quickly through the intestines (diarrhea may be present).

Meat Fibers [Reference range 0 (none seen)]   The presence of microscopic meat fibers are indicators of incomplete protein digestion. There is a correlation between excessive fecal meat fibers and lack or absence of hydrochloric acid secretion (hypochlorhydria and achlorhydria, respectively) and/or insufficient output of pancreatic enzymes.

Vegetable Fibers [Reference range: 0 to 4 fibers]   The presence of an excess of vegetable fibers may be a sign of inadequate chewing more than anything else.

Valerate, iso-Butyrate [Reference range 0 to 10 µm/g]   These compounds are short-chain fatty acids (SCFAs) produced by the bacteria in the gut through breakdown of proteins. In a healthy colon, these specific SCFAs constitute less than 10% of the total concentration of all SCFAs. Higher levels may indicate hypochlorhydria or achlorhydria, and/or insufficient output of pancreatic enzymes.

Absorption

Long-Chain Fatty Acids [Reference range: <1.1%]   These free fatty acids are normally readily absorbed by healthy intestines. In cases of mucosal malabsorption, they accumulate and reach substantial fecal levels. Elevated levels of free fatty acids may reflect malabsorption. Malabsorption may be caused by parasitic infection, inflammatory bowel disease, food allergy, gluten intolerance, and small intestinal bacterial overgrowth.

Cholesterol [Reference range: <0.3%] An elevated cholesterol level in feces is abnormal and usually reflects malabsorption.

Total Fecal Fat [Reference range: <1.6%] This parameter reflects the sum of all fats except the short-chain fatty acids. Elevations may reflect either malabsorption (if long-chain fatty acids are elevated) or impaired digestion (if triglycerides are elevated).

Total Short-Chain Fatty Acids [Reference range: 25 to 155 μm/g] Short-chain fatty acids (SCFAs) are the end products of bacterial breakdown, primarily of carbohydrates. Elevated total levels of the four main SCFAs may reflect malabsorption or bacterial overgrowth. Increased levels also suggest disordered fluid, electrolyte, and acid/base balances of the body. Decreased levels reflect disruption of the normal colonic flora, most often due to antibiotic use.

Colonic Environment

Beneficial Bacteria [Reference range: 2+ to 4+ (within a 0 to 4+ scale)] There are several important resident bacteria that should always be present for optimal intestinal health and function. They are:

Escherichia coli (non-pathogenic resident strain)

Lactobacillus species

Bifidobacteria

These three organisms are cultured and growth is quantitatively measured.

Pathogenic Bacteria The CSDA should also report the presence of bacterial pathogens (disease-causing), by type and amount. Some more common pathogens include:

Aeromonas

Campylobacter

Salmonella

Shigella

Staphylococcus aureus

Vibrio

Yersinia

There are other intestinal bacteria that, while not causing acute gastrointestinal tract disturbances, may be involved in the etiology of various chronic or systemic problems and, through molecular mimicry, in several autoimmune diseases. The presence of any of the following possible pathogens should also be reported:

Klebsiella

Proteus

Pseudomonas

Citrobacter

The CDSA should also report organisms that are characteristic of *imbalanced flora.* It is important to know if bacteria are present that are markers of an imbalanced intestinal ecology. Some bacteria reported in this category include:

Enterobacter

Beta hemolytic Streptococci

Hemolytic E. coli

Hafnia

Mucoid E. coli

Mycology [Reference range: 2+ to 4+ is considered abnormal]   The identification and amount cultured of various yeast species is reported. The common species reported are *C. albicans, C. tropicalis, Rhodotorula,* and *Geotrichum.*

Metabolic Markers

pH [Reference range: 6.0 to 7.2 pH]   There is considerable interest in fecal pH in relation to the risk of colon cancer, especially as affected by fiber intake and the subsequent production of short- and long-chain fatty acids.[4] A correlation between alkaline pH and decreased short-chain fatty acid (particularly butyrate) values has been observed.[5] Clinical studies have also shown a relationship between elevated fecal pH hypochlorhydria. Elevated pH values together with diminished SCFA levels support inadequate bacterial digestion of fiber and/or inadequate intake of dietary fiber.

Short-Chain Fatty Acid Distribution   The amount and proportion of the different short-chain fatty acids reflect the basic health of the intestinal metabolism.[6,7] The most important SCFAs and their proper percentage of the total SCFA are acetate 54% to 67%, proprionate 16% to 24%, and butyrate 14% to 23%. Imbalanced ratios of the SCFA reflect disordered bowel flora (dysbiosis).

Butyrate [Reference range: 10 to 50 μm/gww]   Butyrate is the most important of the SCFAs and is the main energy source for the cells that line the colon (colonic epithelial cells).[8] Adequate amounts are necessary for healthy metabolism and the welfare of the colonic mucosa. Butyrate has been shown to have protective effects against colorectal cancers. Elevated levels are associated with active colitis and inflammatory bowel diseases.

Beta-Glucuronidase [Reference range: 70 to 1,000 IU/g] One of the key ways in which the liver detoxifies cancer-causing chemicals, as well as the body's hormones such as estrogen, is via attaching glucoronic acid to the toxin and excreting it in the bile. Beta-glucuronidase is a bacterial enzyme that uncouples (breaks) the bond between excreted toxins and glucoronic acid. Therefore, the finding that excess beta-glucuronidase activity is associated with an increased cancer risk, particularly estrogen-dependent breast cancer, is not surprising. The activity of this enzyme can be reduced by *lactobacilli* and *bifidobacteria,* reducing meat intake, and increasing dietary fiber intake.

Immunology

Secretory IgA [Reference range: 22 to 140 mcg/g] Secretory IgA (s-IgA) is an antibody secreted by the intestinal lining that acts as the first line of defense in the gastrointestinal tract. Reduced levels of s-IgA mean that the intestinal tract is very susceptible to infection. Reduced levels are commonly seen in food allergies, bacterial overgrowth of the small intestine, chronic candidiasis, and parasitic infections. Elevated levels may reflect an activated immune response to the very same factors that can reduce s-IgA.

Dysbiosis Index [Reference range: <3] The CDSA from Great Smokies comes with a dysbiosis index calculated from all the relevant digestive, metabolic, and microbiological markers. It is often helpful in analyzing the multiple data and provides a quick assessment of the micro-ecology of the gastrointestinal tract.

Macroscopic Observations

Fecal Color [Reference range: light brown to brown] The color of feces is observed and can be indicative of various conditions. Possible indications of abnormality are:

Yellow to green: diarrhea, bowel sterilized by antibiotics

Black: usually the result of upper tract bleeding

Tan or gray: blockage of the common bile duct, severe pancreatic insufficiency (greasy stool), fat malabsorption

Red: possible result of lower tract bleeding

Blood mixed in stool: colonic bleeding (including hemorrhoids)

Mucus [Reference range: absence of mucus] The presence of mucus or pus can be an indication of irritable bowel syndrome, intestinal wall inflammation (caused by infection, e.g., typhoid, *Shigella,* or amoebas), diverticulitis, or other intestinal abscess.

Occult Blood [Reference range: negative] The presence of fecal occult blood represents gastrointestinal tract bleeding. It may be due to something as benign as a hemorrhoid or to something as serious as colon cancer.

Final Comments

Proper digestion is a requirement for optimum health and incomplete or disordered digestion can be a major contributor to the development of many diseases. The problem is not only that ingestion of foods and nutritional substances are of little benefit when breakdown and assimilation are inadequate, but also that incompletely digested food molecules can be inappropriately absorbed into the body. Determining digestive function and assessing the intestinal environment through the CSDA can provide valuable information as to the cause of the disturbance. This information can then be used to restore or achieve improved digestion and a more optimal intestinal environment.

2

Indigestion

The term *indigestion* is often used to describe a feeling of gaseousness or fullness in the abdomen. It can also be used to describe "heartburn." Indigestion can be attributed to a great many causes, including not only increased secretion of acid but also decreased secretion of acid and other digestive factors and enzymes. The dominant treatment of indigestion is the use of over-the-counter preparations. These preparations include antacids, which work by binding free acid, and drugs such as Tagamet, Zantac, and Pepcid, which inhibit the release of hydrochloric-acid antacids by blocking histamine (H2) receptors.

The stomach's optimal pH range is 1.5 to 2.5, with hydrochloric acid being the primary stomach acid. The use of antacids and H2-receptor antagonists typically raises the pH above 3.5. This increase effectively inhibits the action of pepsin, an enzyme involved in protein digestion that can be irritating to the stomach. Although raising the stomach's pH can reduce symptoms, it must be pointed out that hydrochloric acid and pepsin are important factors in protein digestion. If their secretion is insufficient or inhibited, proper protein digestion and mineral disassociation will not occur. In addition, the change in pH can adversely affect gut microbial flora, including the promotion of an overgrowth of *Helicobacter pylori.* Therefore, it is important to use antacids wisely and sparingly. In addition, many nutrition-orientated physicians believe that it is not too much acid but rather a *lack* of acid that is the problem. Typically, in addressing indigestion, naturopathic physicians use measures to enhance rather than inhibit digestion. Commonly used digestive aids include hydrochloric acid and pancreatic enzyme preparations. This chapter will take a critical look at the use of common antacids and other drugs to treat indigestion and contrast their use with enhancing digestion through the use of natural digestive aids.

Heartburn (Reflux Esophagitis)

A 1983 article in the *American Journal of Gastroenterology* asked the question "Why do apparently healthy people use antacids?"[1] The answer: *reflux esophagitis,* the medical term for heartburn. Reflux esophagitis is most often caused by the flow of gastric juices up the esophagus leading to a burning discomfort that radiates upward and is made worse by lying down. Reflux esophagitis is most often caused by overeating. (Remember that old Alka-Seltzer theme? "I can't believe I ate the whole thing.") Other common causes include obesity, cigarette smoking, chocolate, fried foods, carbonated beverages (soft drinks), alcohol, and coffee. These factors either increase the pressure within the stomach, thereby causing the gastric contents to flow upward, or they decrease the tone of the sphincter between the stomach and the esophagus that normally prevents gastric reflux into the esophagus. The first step in treating reflux esophagitis is prevention. In most cases this step simply involves eliminating or reducing the causative factor.

Additional Recommendations for Reflux Esophagitis

For occasional heartburn, antacids may well be appropriate. However, they should not be abused. If heartburn is a chronic problem, it may be a sign of a hiatal hernia, the out-pouching of the stomach above the diaphragm. However, it is interesting to note that while 50% of people over the age of 50 have hiatal hernias, only 5% of patients with hiatal hernias actually experience reflux esophagitis.

Perhaps the most effective treatment of chronic reflux esophagitis and symptomatic hiatal hernias is to utilize gravity. The standard recommendation is to simply place 4-inch blocks under the bedposts at the head of the bed. This elevation of the head is very effective in many cases.

Another recommendation is to heal the esophagus by using deglycyrrhizinated licorice (DGL). Although DGL is primarily used for treating peptic ulcers, I have used it in cases of heartburn with success. DGL is further discussed below and in Chapter 3.

Using Antacids Wisely

All antacids are relatively safe when used on an occasional basis for heartburn or indigestion. Taken regularly, however, they can lead to malabsorption of nutrients, bowel irregularities, kidney stones, and other side effects. There are several types of over-the-counter antacids. Each of these types is discussed below.

Aluminum-Containing Compounds

Aluminum-containing antacids include Maalox, Rolaids, Di-Gel, Mylanta, Riopan, Wingel, Amphogel, and AlternaGEL. Although these antacids are potent and effective in neutralizing acid, there are some significant long-term safety concerns about their use. Ever-growing evidence indicates that aluminum may play a role in impairing mental function as well as in diseases of the nervous system, including Alzheimer's disease, dialysis dementia, Parkinson's disease, and Lou Gehrig's disease (amyotrophic lateral sclerosis).[2-4] Although manufacturers and the FDA tell us that the aluminum in antacids is not absorbed, this appears to be fraudulent information as absorption studies prove otherwise even when low-dose therapy is used.[5-7] Absorption of aluminum is greatly enhanced if the meal contains any citrus fruit, orange juice, soda pop, or other source of citric acid. The bottom line is that there is no reason to use the aluminum-containing antacids at this time as the potential risk far outweighs the short-term benefit.

Sodium Bicarbonate

Sodium bicarbonate is baking soda. Alka-Seltzer is simply ordinary baking soda in an effervescent form. Although sodium bicarbonate can be useful in short-term therapy, it is not indicated for chronic or prolonged therapy due to the risk of sodium overload. In addition, because the bicarbonate ion is rapidly absorbed, long-term administration can cause systemic alkalosis (excessive pH throughout the body). This can lead to the formation of kidney stones, nausea, vomiting, headaches, and mental confusion.

Calcium Carbonate and Calcium Citrate

An example of a calcium carbonate-containing antacid is Tums. Although fast-acting and potent, calcium carbonate can produce what is known as "acid rebound" three or four hours after use. This means that the body will try to overcompensate the neutralization of gastric acid by secreting even more acid. This is not viewed as being clinically significant in the treatment of indigestion, but it may play a role in delaying ulcer healing.

Many physicians recommend Tums as a calcium supplement. In fact, calcium carbonate is the most widely used form of calcium supplement. While calcium carbonate is an effective antacid, there are better forms of calcium for supplementation.

In order for calcium carbonate and other insoluble calcium salts to be assimilated, they must first be solubilized and ionized by stomach acid. This is where the problem arises with calcium carbonate for many individuals. In studies with postmenopausal women, it has been shown that about 40% are severely deficient in stomach acid.[8] It has been shown that patients with insufficient stomach acid output can only absorb about 4% of an oral dose of calcium as calcium carbonate while a person with normal stomach acid can typically absorb about 22%.[9] Patients with low stomach acid secretion need a form of calcium already in a soluble and ionized state, like calcium bound to Krebs cycle intermediates (e.g., citrate, malate, succinate, and fumarate) or lactate and aspartate. About 45% of the calcium is absorbed from calcium citrate in patients with reduced stomach acid compared to 4% absorption for calcium carbonate. It has also been demonstrated that calcium is more bioavailable from calcium citrate than from calcium carbonate in normal subjects as well.[10]

The strong alkaline nature of carbonate, combined with the calcium that is absorbed, greatly increases the risk of kidney stones, especially if milk products are a regular part of the diet. In contrast, the chemical nature of citrate actually prevents kidney stones from developing.[11] This, along with its superior absorption, clearly demonstrates that calcium citrate is much more beneficial than calcium car-bonate as a calcium supplement.

In addition, calcium citrate may be the best antacid as well. Calcium citrate has shown impressive results as an antacid (phosphate binder) in patients with kidney disease.[12] It is much better tolerated than aluminum-containing antacids. Although I am not aware of any calcium-citrate preparations being marketed as antacids, preparations of calcium citrate and calcium bound to other Krebs-cycle intermediates are widely available.

Magnesium Compounds

Magnesium salts, such as magnesium oxide, hydroxide, and carbonate, often appear in aluminum-containing products. Phillip's Milk of Magnesia is the only major brand that features only magnesium; it is a suspension of magnesium hydroxide in water. In addition to acting as a mild antacid, magnesium hydroxide also exerts a laxative effect. It is a safe and effective product for people with normal kidney function, although diarrhea is a definite risk.

H2-Receptor Antagonists

These drugs work to block the action of histamine on the secretion of stomach acid. Histamine stimulates the secretion of stomach acid. By blocking this effect of histamine, stomach acid output is greatly reduced. Examples of H2-receptor antagonists include cimitidine (Tagamet), raniti-dine (Zantac), famotidine (Pepcid), and nizatidine (Axid).

Recently the makers of these drugs were able to encourage the FDA to make them available over the counter. As a result, I believe we may see more problems with digestive disturbances and other side effects caused by these drugs. Since H2-receptor antagonists block a vital bodily function involved in digestion, digestive disturbances are quite common and can include nausea, constipation, and diarrhea. Nutrient deficiencies can appear as a result of impaired digestion. Other possible side effects include bacterial overgrowth (including overgrowth of *Helicobacter pylori*), liver damage, allergic reactions, headaches, breast enlargement in men, hair loss, osteoporosis, dizziness, depression, insomnia, and impotence.

The Natural Approach to Indigestion

Although some antacids are in essence natural products and have an appropriate use in treating occasional indigestion, in most chronic cases a more critical look at the problem of indigestion is needed. In the patient with chronic indigestion, rather than focus on blocking the digestive process with antacids, the natural approach to indigestion focuses on aiding digestion.

Although much is said about hyperacidity conditions, probably a more common cause of indigestion is a lack of gastric acid secretion. Hypochlorhydria refers to deficient gastric acid secretion while achlorhydria refers to a complete absence of gastric acid secretion.

There are many symptoms and signs that suggest impaired gastric acid secretion, and a number of specific diseases have been found to be associated with insufficient gastric acid output.[13–24] These are listed in Tables 2.1 and 2.2.

Several studies have shown that the ability to secrete gastric acid decreases with age.[25–27] Some studies found low stomach acidity in over half of those over age 60. The best method of diagnosing a lack of gastric acid is a special procedure known as the *Heidelberg gastric analysis*.[28] This technique utilizes an electronic capsule attached to a string. The capsule is swallowed and then kept in the stomach with the aid of the string. The capsule measures

Table 2.1   Common Signs and Symptoms of
Low Gastric Acidity

Bloating, belching, burning, and flatulence immediately after meals
A sense of "fullness" after eating
Indigestion, diarrhea, or constipation
Multiple food allergies
Nausea after taking supplements
Itching around the rectum
Weak, peeling, and cracked fingernails
Dilated blood vessels in the cheeks and nose
Acne
Iron deficiency
Chronic intestinal parasites or abnormal flora
Undigested food in stool
Chronic candida infections
Upper digestive tract gassiness

the pH of the stomach and sends a radio message to a receiver, which then records the pH level. Dr. Jonathan Wright believes the response to a bicarbonate challenge during Heidelberg gastric analysis is the true test of the functional ability of the stomach to secrete acid.[29] After the test, the capsule is pulled up from the stomach by the string attached to it.

Since not everyone can have detailed gastric acid analysis to determine the need for gastric acid supplementation, a more practical method of determination is often used. If an individual is experiencing any signs and symptoms of gastric acid insufficiency as listed above in Table 2.1 or has any of the diseases listed in Table 2.2, the method outlined below can be employed to determine gastric acid sufficiency.

Table 2.2   Diseases Associated with Low Gastric Acidity

Addison's disease
Asthma
Celiac disease
Dermatitis herpetiformis
Diabetes mellitus
Eczema
Gallbladder disease
Graves' disease
Chronic autoimmune disorders
Hepatitis
Chronic hives
Lupus erythematosis
Myasthenia gravis
Osteoporosis
Pernicious anemia
Psoriasis
Rheumatoid arthritis
Rosacea
Sjogren's syndrome
Thyrotoxicosis
Hyper- and hypothyroidism
Vitiligo

Protocol for Hydrochloric Acid Supplements

1. Begin by taking one tablet or capsule containing 10 grains (600 mg) of hydrochloric acid (HCl) at your next large meal. If this does not aggravate your symptoms, at every meal after that of the same size take one additional tablet or capsule.(Two at the next meal, three at the meal after that, then four at the next meal . . .)

2. Continue to increase the dose until you reach seven tablets or you feel a warmth in your stomach, whichever occurs first. A feeling of warmth in the stomach means that you have taken too many tablets for that meal and you need to take one less tablet for that size of meal. It is a good idea to try the larger dose again at another meal to make sure that it was the HCl that caused the warmth and not something else.

3. After you have found the largest dose that you can take at your large meals without feeling any warmth, maintain that dose at all your meals of similar size. You will need to take less at smaller meals.

4. When taking a number of tablets or capsules, it is best to take them throughout the meal.

5. As your stomach begins to regain the ability to produce the amount of HCl needed to properly digest your food, you will notice the warm feeling again and will have to cut down the dose level.

What Causes Hypochlorhydria?

Like peptic ulcer disease (discussed in Chapter 3), achlorhydria and hypochlorhydria have been linked to the overgrowth of the bacteria *Helicobacter pylori.* It has been shown that 90% to 100% of patients with duodenal ulcers, 70% with gastric ulcers, and about 50% of people over the age of 50 test positive for *H. pylori.*[30] The presence of *H. pylori* is established by determining the level of antibodies to *H. pylori* in the blood or saliva, or by culturing material collected during an endoscopy (examining the stomach with a tubelike instrument with a lens attached) as well as measuring the breath for urea.

Low gastric output is thought to predispose one to *H. pylori* colonization and *H. pylori* colonization increases gastric pH, thereby setting up a positive feedback scenario and increasing the likelihood of the colonization of the stomach and duodenum with other organisms.[31] Interestingly, there has been only scant research into the effects of antacids and H2-receptor antagonists on promoting *H. pylori* overgrowth.[32]

If *H. pylori* gastritis leads to achlorhydria, the next obvious question is, What are the factors that lead to *H. pylori* gastritis? Consistent with history, conventional medicine is obsessed with the infective agent rather than host defense factors. This obsession began with Louis Pasteur, the nineteenth-century physician and researcher who discovered the antibiotic effects of penicillin. Pasteur played a major role in the development of the germ theory. This theory holds that different diseases are caused by different infectious organisms. Much of Pasteur's life was dedicated to finding substances that would kill the infecting organisms. Pasteur and others since him who've pioneered effective treatments of infectious diseases have given us a great deal, for which we all should be thankful. However, there is more to the equation than the virility of the infectious organism.

Another nineteenth-century French scientist, Claude Bernard, also made major contributions to medical understanding. However, Bernard had a different view of health and disease. Bernard believed that the state of a person's internal environment or *milieu interieur* was more important in determining disease than the organism or pathogen itself. In other words, Bernard believed that the internal "terrain" or host susceptibility to infection was more important than the germ. Physicians, he believed, should focus more of their attention on making this internal terrain an inhospitable place for disease to flourish.

Bernard's theory led to some rather interesting studies. In fact, a firm advocate of the germ theory would find some of these studies to be absolutely crazy. One of the most interesting studies was conducted by a Russian scientist named Elie Metchnikoff, the discoverer of the white blood cells. He and his research associates consumed cultures containing millions of cholera bacteria. Yet none of them developed cholera. The reason: Their immune systems were not compromised. Metchnikoff believed, like Bernard, that the correct way to deal with infectious disease was to focus on enhancing the body's own defenses.

During the last part of their lives, Pasteur and Bernard engaged in scientific discussions on the virtues of the germ theory versus Bernard's perspective on the internal terrain. On his deathbed, Pasteur said: "Bernard was right. The pathogen is nothing. The terrain is everything."

Unfortunately, Pasteur's legacy is the conventional medical profession's obsession with the pathogen; modern medicine has largely forgotten the importance of the "terrain."

Treating *H. Pylori* Overgrowth Naturally

Unfortunately, because most research focuses on eradicating the organism, there is little information on protective factors against infectivity. Proposed protective factors against *H. pylori*-induced intestinal damage are maintaining a low pH and ensuring adequate antioxidant defense mechanisms.[33-35] Low levels of vitamin C, vitamin E, and other antioxidant factors in the gastric juice appear not only to lead to the progression of *H. pylori* colonization, but also contribute to the ulcer-causing potential of *H. pylori*.[36] Not everyone infected with *H. pylori* gets peptic ulcer disease or gastric cancer. Those most susceptible to these diseases appear to have inadequate levels of anti-oxidants as well as inadequate gastric acid output.

Deglycyrrhizinated Licorice

As for how to eradicate the organism as well as stimulate increased host defense factors, I recommend deglycyrrhizinated licorice (DGL). DGL has shown good results in healing both duodenal ulcers and gastric ulcers (discussed more fully on page 40). Rather than inhibit the release of acid, DGL stimulates the normal defense mechanisms that prevent ulcer formation. Specifically, DGL improves both the quality and quantity of the protective substances that line the intestinal tract; increases the life span of the intestinal cell; and improves blood supply to the intestinal lining.[37,38] Numerous clinical studies over the years have found DGL to be an effective anti-ulcer compound. In several head-to-head comparison studies, DGL has been shown to be more effective than Tagamet, Zantac, or antacids in both short-term treatment and maintenance therapy of peptic ulcers.[39-42]

The active components of DGL are believed to be special flavonoid derivatives. These compounds have demonstrated impressive protection against chemically-induced ulcer formation in animal studies. Does DGL have any effect on *Helicobacter pylori?* The answer appears to be yes. In a recent study, several flavonoids were shown to inhibit *H. pylori* in a clear-cut concentration-dependent manner.[43] In addition, unlike antibiotics, the flavonoids also augment natural defense factors that prevent ulcer formation. The activity of flavone, the most potent flavonoid in the study, was shown to be similar to that of bismuth subcitrate (discussed on page 30).

In order to be effective in healing peptic ulcers, it appears that DGL must mix with saliva. DGL may promote the release of salivary compounds that stimulate the growth and regeneration of stomach and intestinal cells. DGL in capsule form has not been shown to be effective. The standard dosage for DGL is two to four 380 mg chewable tablets between or 20 minutes before meals. Taking DGL after meals is associated with poor results.[44] DGL therapy should be continued for at least 8 to 16 weeks after there is a full therapeutic response.

Bismuth Subcitrate

Bismuth is a naturally occurring mineral that can act as an antacid as well as exert activity against *H. pylori*. The best known and most widely used bismuth preparation is bismuth subsalicylate (Pepto-Bismol). However, bismuth subcitrate has produced the best results against *H. pylori* and in the treatment of non-ulcer related indigestion as well as peptic ulcers.[45,46] In the United States, bismuth subcitrate preparations are available through compounding pharmacies (to find a compounding pharmacist in your area, call the International Academy of Compounding Pharmacists 1-800-927-4227).

One of the key advantages of bismuth preparations over standard antibiotic approaches to eradicating *H. pylori* is that while the bacteria may develop resistance to various antibiotics it is very unlikely to develop resistance to bismuth.

The usual dosage for bismuth subcitrate is 240 mg twice daily before meals. For bismuth subsalicylate the dosage is 500 mg (two tablets or 30 ml of standard strength Pepto-Bismol) four times daily.

Bismuth preparations are extremely safe when taken at prescribed dosages. Bismuth subcitrate may cause a temporary and harmless darkening of the tongue and/or stool. Bismuth subsalicylate should not be taken by children recovering from the flu, chicken pox, or some other viral infection, because it may mask the nausea and vomiting associated with Reye's syndrome, a rare but serious illness.

Pancreatic Enzymes as Digestive Aids

Nutrition-oriented physicians use both physical symptoms and laboratory tests to assess pancreatic function. Common symptoms of pancreatic insufficiency include abdominal bloating and discomfort, gas, indigestion, and the passing of undigested food in the stool. For laboratory diagnosis, most nutrition-oriented physicians use the comprehensive stool and digestive analysis (see page 6).

Pancreatic insufficiency is characterized by impaired digestion, malabsorption, nutrient deficiencies, and abdominal discomfort. The most severe level of pancreatic insufficiency is seen in cystic fibrosis, an inherited disorder. Although cystic fibrosis is quite rare, mild pancreatic insufficiency is thought to be a relatively common condition, especially in the elderly.

Pancreatic enzyme products are the most effective treatment for pancreatic insufficiency and are also quite popular digestive aids. Most commercial preparations are prepared from fresh hog pancreas (pancreatin).

The dosage of pancreatic enzymes is based on the level of enzyme activity of the particular product. The United States Pharmacopoeia (USP) has set strict definitions for level of activity. A 1X pancreatic enzyme (pancreatin) product has in each milligram not less than 25 USP units of amylase activity, not less than 2.0 USP units of lipase activity, and not less than 25 USP units for protease activity. Pancreatin of higher potency is given a whole number multiple indicating its strength. For example, a full-strength undiluted pancreatic extract that is 10 times stronger than the USP standard would be referred to as 10X USP. Full-strength products are preferred to lower potency pancreatin products because lower potency products are often diluted with salt, lactose, or galactose to achieve desired strength (e.g., 4X or 1X). The dosage recommendation for a 10X USP pancreatic enzyme product would be 350 to 1,000 mg, three times a day immediately before meals when used as a digestive aid and 10 to 20 minutes before meals or on an empty stomach when antiinflammatory effects are desired.

Enzyme products are often enteric-coated, that is they are often coated to prevent digestion in the stomach, so that the enzymes will be liberated in the small intestine. However, numerous studies have shown that non-enteric-coated enzyme preparations actually outperform enteric-coated products if they are given prior to a meal (for digestive purposes) or on an empty stomach (for anti-inflammatory effects).

For vegetarians, bromelain and papain (protein-digesting enzymes from pineapple and papaya, respectively) can substitute for pancreatic enzymes in the treatment of pancreatic insufficiency, however, in my experience, the best results are obtained if they are used in combination with pancreatin and ox bile.

Pancreatin in Preventing Food Allergies

While starch and fat digestion can be carried out satisfactorily without the help of pancreatic enzymes, the proteases are critical to proper protein digestion. Incomplete digestion of proteins creates a number of problems for the body including the development of food allergies.

In order for a food molecule to produce an allergic response, it must be a fairly large molecule. In studies performed in the 1930s and 1940s, pancreatic enzymes were shown to be quite effective in preventing food allergies.[47] It appears that many practitioners are not aware of or perhaps they have forgotten about these early studies. Typically individuals who do not secrete enough proteases will suffer from multiple food allergies.

Final Comments

Although antacids and H2-receptor antagonists may lead to relief of symptoms attributed to indigestion, they actually interfere with the digestive process and disrupt gut microbial ecology. A better approach is to enhance digestion with the help of digestive aids such as hydrochloric acid, pancreatin, and enzyme preparations. A complete stool and digestive analysis can be invaluable for helping to determine which digestive aid will work best, but even so, it usually comes down to trial and error. The digestive system is a true system. Affecting any single component of the system generally affects the entire system.

3

Peptic Ulcers

When somebody says they have an ulcer, they are usually referring to a *peptic ulcer*. The most common locations for peptic ulcer formation are in the stomach (gastric ulcer) and the first portion of the small intestine (duodenal ulcer). Although duodenal and gastric ulcers occur at different locations, they appear to be the result of similar mechanisms. Specifically, the development of a peptic ulcer is the result of some factor damaging the protective factors that line the stomach and duodenum.

In the past, the medical establishment has focused primarily on the acidic secretions of the stomach as the primary cause of both gastric and duodenal ulcers. However, more recently the focus has been on the bacteria *H. pylori* (see page 26).

The acid secreted by the stomach is strong enough to burn your skin and produce an ulcer. So how do the stomach and duodenum protect against ulcer formation? There are actually several important ways including the production of a mucus, which lines and protects against ulcer formation; the constant renewing of intestinal cells; and the secretion of factors that neutralize the acid when it comes in contact with the stomach and intestinal linings.

Under normal circumstances, there are enough protective factors to prevent ulcer formation, however, when there is a decrease in the integrity of these protective factors, an ulcer can form. A loss of integrity can be the result of alcohol, drugs (particularly drugs used in arthritis), nutrient deficiency, stress, *H. pylori* infection, and many other factors.

Although symptoms of a peptic ulcer may be absent or quite vague, most peptic ulcers are associated with abdominal discomfort, usually noted 45 to 60 minutes after meals or during the night. In a typical case, the pain is described as gnawing, burning, cramp-like, or aching, or as "heartburn." Eating or using antacids usually results in great relief.

Individuals with any symptoms of a peptic ulcer need competent medical care. Peptic-ulcer complications such as hemorrhage, perforation, and obstruction represent medical emergencies that require immediate hospitalization. Individuals with peptic ulcers should be monitored by a physician, even if following the natural approaches discussed below.

Peptic Ulcer Medications

Medical treatment of peptic ulcers focuses on reducing gastric acidity with antacids and drugs that block stomach acid secretion (H2-receptor antagonists—see page 22.) In addition to this standard drug approach, eradicating *H. pylori* with antibiotics is quickly becoming part of the ulcer treatment regimen.

Perhaps the most popular regimen being prescribed by most allopathic (traditional) medical doctors is the so-called "triple-drug therapy," consisting of tetracycline, bismuth subsalicylate, and metronidazole in combination with an H2-receptor antagonist such as Tagamet or Zantac. This approach has produced better results compared to using antacids or H2-receptor antagonists alone, but it carries with it some risk of side effects and the likelihood that the bacteria may build up a resistance to the antibiotic.

Whether *H. pylori* is a direct cause or simply a contributor to ulcer formation has not yet been determined. What is known is that *H. pylori* can be found in 70% to 75% of gastric ulcers and 90% to 100% of duodenal ulcers.[1] *H. pylori* is thought to contribute to peptic ulcers by burrowing itself into the junction between the intestinal cells and then secreting an enzyme that breaks down the mucus which protects the intestinal lining. Indigestion, inflammation, and ulceration can follow.

The Natural Approach to Peptic Ulcers

The natural approach to treating peptic ulcers is to first identify and then eliminate or reduce all factors that can contribute to the development of peptic ulcers: food allergy, low-fiber diet, cigarette smoking, stress, alcohol, and drugs (especially aspirin and other non-steroidal anti-inflammatory drugs). Once the causative factors have been controlled or eliminated, the focus is directed at healing the ulcers and promoting tissue resistance. As discussed on page 27, rather than focus on the invading organism, naturopathic physicians choose to focus on the terrain. A highly nutritious diet and a health-promoting lifestyle go a long way in making the terrain less hospitable to *H. pylori* and thus preventing peptic ulcers. These factors and the use of selected nutrients, cabbage juice, and deglycyrrhizinated licorice will be described below.

A Fiber-Rich Diet

A diet rich in fiber is both preventive and therapeutic.[2] This is probably a result of fiber's ability to promote a healthy protective layer of mucin in the stomach and intestines as well as act as a buffering agent. Although several fibers often used to supplement the diet (e.g., pectin, guar gum, psyllium, etc.) have been shown to produce beneficial effects[3,4], it is best to simply eat a diet rich in plant foods (see Chapter 7).

Food Allergies

There is much evidence pointing to food allergy as a prime causative factor of peptic ulcers.[5] In addition, a diet eliminating food allergies has been used with great success in treating and preventing recurrent ulcers.[6] Food allergy may explain the high recurrence rate of peptic ulcers. If food allergy is the cause, the ulcer will continue to recur until the allergenic food has been eliminated from the diet.

It is ironic that many people with peptic ulcers soothe themselves by consuming milk, a highly allergenic food. Milk should be avoided on this basis alone. Additional evidence suggests that milk should be particularly avoided in patients with peptic ulcers; population studies have shown that the higher the milk consumption, the greater the likelihood of ulcers. In addition, milk significantly increases stomach acid production.[7]

Smoking

Increased frequency of peptic ulcers, decreased response to peptic-ulcer therapy, and an increased mortality due to peptic ulcers are all related to smoking. Three postulated mechanisms for this association are decreased pancreatic bicarbonate secretion (an important neutralizer of gastric acid), increased reflux of bile salts into the stomach, and acceleration of gastric emptying into the duodenum. Bile salts are extremely irritating to the stomach and initial portions of the duodenum. Bile salt reflux induced by smoking appears to be the most likely factor responsible for the increased peptic ulcer rate in smokers. However, the psychological aspects of smoking also are important, since the chronic anxiety and psychological stress associated with smoking appear to worsen ulcer activity.

Stress and Emotional Factors

Stress is universally believed to be an important factor in the development of peptic ulcers. However, this belief is based on uncontrolled observations; and in the medical literature the role of stress in the development of peptic ulcers is controversial.

Several studies have shown that the number of stressful life events is not significantly different in peptic-ulcer patients as compared to carefully selected, ulcer-free controls, but this finding doesn't hold much significance because it is not simply the amount of stress that is important to consider. What is important is an individual's response to stress. Two people can experience the same stressful situation, yet handle it in completely different manners. Ulcer patients have been characterized as tending to repress their emotions rather than express what they are feeling. Learning to deal with stress and the expression of emotions is critical to long-term health.

Selected Nutrients

Numerous individual nutrients are important to the health of the stomach and intestinal lining. Most important are vitamins A, C, and E, and zinc.[8] These nutrients have been shown to inhibit the development of ulcers in laboratory animals and several clinical studies have shown a positive therapeutic effect as well. Rather than taking each of these nutrients separately, it may be best to simply take a good multiple vitamin-mineral preparation.

Cabbage Juice

Cabbage juice was shown to be extremely effective in the treatment of peptic ulcers by Dr. Garnett Cheney of Stanford University's School of Medicine and other researchers in the 1950s.[9,10] Cheney believed that cabbage juice contained a substance he called "vitamin U" (the U stood for ulcer). Although this factor was never clearly identified, Cheney clearly demonstrated that fresh cabbage juice is extremely effective in the treatment of peptic ulcers, usually in less than seven days. Here is one of Dr. Cheney's favorite cabbage juice recipes:

Dr. Cheney's Vitamin U Drink

½ head or 2 cups of green cabbage
1 to 2 tomatoes
4 ribs of celery
2 carrots

Cut the cabbage (green cabbages are best) into long wedges and feed through the juicer, followed by the tomatoes, then the celery and carrots. Drink twice daily for as long as ulcer symptoms are present.

Deglycyrrhizinated Licorice

A special licorice extract known as deglycyrrhizinated licorice (DGL) is a remarkable anti-ulcer agent (it is briefly described on page 29).[11,12] DGL is produced by concentrating licorice for glycyrrhetinic acid and then removing this compound. Glycyrrhetinic acid and crude licorice preparations can cause elevations in blood pressure due to high levels of sodium, causing water retention. DGL, however, is free of side effects.

Numerous studies over the years have found DGL to be an effective anti-ulcer compound. In several head-to-head comparison studies, DGL has been shown to be more effective than Tagamet, Zantac, or antacids in both short-term treatment and maintenance therapy of peptic ulcers.[13,14] In addition, while these drugs are associated with significant side effects, DGL is extremely safe and is only a fraction of the cost. For example, while Tagamet and Zantac typically cost well over $100 for a month's supply, DGL is available in health food stores at $15.00 for a month's supply.

Using DGL with Gastric Ulcers

In a study using DGL to treat gastric ulcers, 33 gastric-ulcer patients were treated with either DGL (760 mg, three times a day) or a placebo for one month.[15] There was a significantly greater reduction in ulcer size in the DGL group (78%), than in the placebo group (34%). Complete healing occurred in 44% of those receiving DGL, but in only 6% of the placebo group.

Subsequent studies have shown DGL to be as effective as Tagamet and Zantac for both short-term treatment and maintenance therapy for gastric ulcers. For example, in a head-to-head comparison with Tagamet, 100 patients received either DGL (760 mg, three times a day between meals) or Tagamet (200 mg, three times a day and 400 mg at bedtime).[13] The percentage of ulcers healed after 6 and 12 weeks were similar in both groups. Yet while Tagamet is associated with some toxicity (see page 22), DGL is extremely safe to use.

Gastric ulcers are often a result of the use of alcohol, aspirin and other non-steroidal anti-inflammatory drugs, caffeine, and other factors that decrease the integrity of the gastric lining. As DGL has been shown to reduce the gastric bleeding caused by aspirin, DGL is strongly indicated for the prevention of gastric ulcers in patients requiring long-term treatment with ulcerogenic drugs, such as aspirin, non-steroidal anti-inflammatory agents, and corticosteroids.[16]

Using DGL with Duodenal Ulcers

DGL is also effective in treating duodenal ulcers. In one study of 40 patients with chronic duodenal ulcers of 4 to 12 years' duration and more than six relapses during the previous year were treated with DGL.[12] All of the patients had been referred for surgery because of relentless pain, sometimes with frequent vomiting, despite treatment with bed rest, antacids, and anticholinergic drugs. Half of the patients received 3 grams of DGL daily for 8 weeks; the other half received 4.5 grams per day for 16 weeks. All 40 patients showed substantial improvement, usually within five to seven days, and none required surgery during the one year follow-up. Although both dosages were effective, the higher dose was significantly more effective than the lower dose.

In another more recent study, the therapeutic effect of DGL was compared to that of antacids or cimetidine in 874 patients with confirmed chronic duodenal ulcers.[14] Ninety-one percent of all the ulcers healed within 12 weeks; there was no significant difference in healing rate in the groups. However, there were fewer relapses in the DGL group (8.2%) than in those receiving cimetidine (12.9%), or antacids (16.4%). These results, coupled with DGL's protective effects, suggest that DGL is a superior treatment for duodenal ulcers.

Dosage Instructions for DGL

In order to be effective in healing peptic ulcers, it appears that DGL must mix with saliva. DGL may promote the release of salivary compounds that stimulate the growth and regeneration of stomach and intestinal cells. The standard dose for DGL is two to four 380 mg chewable tablets, between or 20 minutes before meals. DGL should be continued for 8 to 16 weeks after cessation of symptoms to ensure complete healing. DGL is available at health food stores.

Final Comments

I believe the natural approach to peptic ulcers is clearly superior to the current medical treatment because it addresses the cause of most people's ulcers—a lack of factors that protect against ulcer development. Here is a concise recommendation that I give my patients with ulcers:

1. Eliminate sugar and refined carbohydrates such as white flour from your diet.
2. Eliminate milk and eggs from your diet.
3. Increase your consumption of whole grains, legumes, and vegetables.
4. Get a juicer and drink 16 to 24 ounces of vegetable juice per day, including the regular consumption of cabbage juice.
5. Take a high-potency multiple vitamin-mineral formula with meals.
6. Take two tablets that contain 380 mg of DGL, 20 minutes before meals.

4

Small Intestine Disturbances

The small intestine is the primary site for absorption of nutrients. While you may think of the small intestine (and the entire digestive tract for that matter) as a simple cylinder, its absorptive surface is composed of microscopic finger-like projections known as *villi* and smaller microvilli attached to the villi. If the entire surface area of the small intestine were spread out flat, it would extend nearly two tennis courts.

One of the small intestine's vital roles is in the distinction of whether to absorb a molecule or act as a barrier to keep it from being absorbed. While our body requires the nutrients contained within the small intestine, it certainly does not desire bacteria, toxic metabolites, and other toxins. It is the role of the small intestine to distinguish whether or not a substance should be granted entry.

This chapter will discuss four conditions that disturb small intestine function—celiac disease (gluten intolerance), small intestine bacterial overgrowth, candidiasis, and the leaky gut syndrome.

Celiac Disease

Celiac disease, also known as non-tropical sprue, gluten-sensitive enteropathy, or celiac sprue, is characterized by malabsorption and an abnormal small intestine structure that reverts to normal on removal of dietary gluten. The protein gluten and its polypeptide derivative, gliadin, are found primarily in wheat, barley, and rye grains.

Symptoms of celiac disease most commonly appear during the first three years of life, after cereals are introduced into the diet. A second peak incidence occurs during the third decade of life. Breast feeding appears to have preventive effects; breast-fed babies have a decreased risk of developing celiac disease.[1-3]

The early introduction of cow's milk is believed to be a major causative factor in the development of celiac disease.[1-4] Research in the past few years has clearly indicated that breast feeding, along with delayed administration of cow's milk and cereal grains, are primary preventive steps that can greatly reduce the risk of developing celiac disease.

Celiac disease also appears to have a genetic cause.[3,5] The frequency of individuals having the genetic trait for celiac disease is much higher in northern and central Europe and the northwest Indian subcontinent.[3,6] Wheat cultivation in these areas is a relatively recent development (1000 B.C.). The prevalence of celiac disease is much higher in these areas compared with other parts of the world (e.g., 1:300 in southwest Ireland compared with 1:2,500 in the United States).

Diagnostic Summary

Celiac disease is a chronic intestinal malabsorption disorder caused by an intolerance to gluten. Symptoms include:

Bulky, pale, frothy, foul-smelling, greasy stools with increased fecal fat

Weight loss and signs of multiple vitamin and mineral deficiencies

Increased levels of serum gliadin antibodies

Diagnosis confirmed by jejunal biopsy

Treatment of Celiac Disease

Once the diagnosis has been established, a gluten-free diet is indicated. This diet does not contain any wheat, rye, barley, triticale, or oats. Rice and corn are generally not a problem while buckwheat and millet are often excluded. Although buckwheat is not in the grass family, and millet appears to be more closely related to rice and corn, they do contain compounds with similar structures to wheat gluten. In addition, milk and milk products should also be eliminated.

Maintenance of a strict gluten-free diet is quite difficult in the United States, due to the wide distribution of gliadin and other activators of celiac disease in processed foods. Individuals with celiac disease must be encouraged to read labels carefully in order to avoid hidden sources of gliadin, such as is found in some brands of soy sauce, modified food starch, ice cream, soup, beer, wine, vodka, whisky, malt, and so on.

Usually clinical improvement will be apparent within a few days or weeks (30% respond within three days, another 50% within one month, and 10% within another month). However, 10% of patients respond only after 24 to 36 months of gluten avoidance.

Resources for Those with Celiac Disease

If you have celiac disease, here is a list of helpful organizations to contact:

American Celiac Society
45 Gifford Avenue
Jersey City, NJ 07304

American Digestive Disease Society
7720 Wisconsin Avenue
Bethesda, MD 20014

Gluten Intolerance Group of North America
P.O. Box 23053
Seattle, WA 98102

National Digestive Disease Education and Information
Clearing House
1555 Wilson Boulevard, Suite 600
Rosslyn, VA 22209

Additional Recommendations

If an individual with celiac disease does not appear to be responding, the following should be considered: (1) incorrect diagnosis, (2) the patient is not adhering to the diet or is being exposed to hidden sources of gliadin, and/or (3) the presence of an associated disease or complication, such as zinc deficiency.[3,7] The latter highlights the importance of multivitamin and mineral supplementation in these patients. In addition to treating any underlying deficiency, supplementation provides the necessary cofactors for growth and repair. Celiac disease will be unresponsive to dietary therapy if an underlying zinc deficiency is present.

Papain, the protein-digesting enzyme from papaya, has been shown to digest wheat gluten and render it harmless in celiac disease subjects.[8] Taking a papain supplement (500 to 1,000 mg) with meals may allow some individuals to tolerate gluten.[9]

Pancreatic enzyme supplementation during the month following the initial diagnosis of celiac disease appears to be worthwhile according to the results of a recent study.

The double-blind study sought to clarify the benefit of pancreatic enzyme therapy because previous studies had shown pancreatic insufficiency in 8% to 30% of celiac patients. In the study, patients followed a gluten-free diet and received either two capsules of pancreatic enzymes with each meal (6 to 10 capsules a day with each capsule containing lipase 5,000 IU, amylase 2,900 IU, and protease 330 IU) or two placebo capsules with meals. Complete nutritional evaluations were conducted at day 0, 30, and 60. Results indicated that pancreatic enzyme supplementation enhanced the clinical benefit of a gluten-free diet during the first 30 days, but did not provide any greater benefit than the placebo after 60 days. These results support the use of pancreatic enzyme preparations in the first 30 days after diagnosis of celiac disease.[10]

Small Intestinal Bacterial Overgrowth

The upper portion of the human small intestine is designed to be relatively free of bacteria. The reason is simple—when bacteria are present in significant concentrations in the duodenum and jejunum, they compete with their host (the human body) for nutrition. When bacteria (or yeast) get to the food first, problems can occur. The organism can ferment the carbohydrates and produce excessive gas, bloating, and abdominal distention. If that is not bad enough, the bacteria can also break down protein via the process of putrefaction to produce what are known as *vasoactive amines.*[11]

For example, bacteria and yeast contain enzymes (decarboxylases) that can convert the amino acid histidine to histamine and tyrosine to tyramine. Compounds produced from the amino acids ornithine and lysine are the dangerous sounding putrescine and cadaverine, respectively. All of these compounds are termed *vasoactive amines* to signify their ability to cause constriction and relaxation of blood vessels by acting on the smooth muscle that surrounds the vessels. In the intestinal tract, excessive vasoactive amine synthesis can lead to increased gut permeability (i.e., the leaky gut syndrome, which is discussed later in this chapter), abdominal pain, and altered gut motility.

Diagnosis of small intestinal bacterial overgrowth involves careful evaluation of the comprehensive digestive and stool analysis. Breath tests that measure the levels of hydrogen and methane after the administration of carbohydrates (lactulose and glucose) also can be used to detect bacterial overgrowth in the small intestine. If there is small intestinal bacterial overgrowth, there will be higher than normal amounts of hydrogen and/or methane.

Symptoms of small intestinal bacterial overgrowth are similar to those generally attributed to achlorhydria and pancreatic insufficiency—namely, indigestion and a sense of fullness (bloating)—but they may also include symptoms generally associated with candida overgrowth (discussed on page 53), more severe gastrointestinal symptoms such as nausea and diarrhea, and arthritis. A study published in the *Annals of the Rheumatic Diseases* in 1993 demonstrated that many patients with rheumatoid arthritis exhibit small intestinal bacterial overgrowth, which was associated with the severity of symptoms and disease activity.[12]

Underlying Causes of Bacterial Overgrowth

The digestive secretions—in particular, hydrochloric acid, bile, and pancreatic enzymes—play a critical role in preventing significant numbers of bacteria from migrating up the small intestine.[13-15] Thus, deficiencies of these secretions can result in bacterial overgrowth (see Table 4.1).

Table 4.1 Factors Associated with
Small Intestinal Bacterial Overgrowth

Decreased digestive secretions
Achlorhydria
Hypochlorhydria
Drugs that inhibit hydrochloric acid
Pancreatic insufficiency
Decreased bile output due to liver or gallbladder disease

Decreased motility
Scleroderma (progressive systemic sclerosis)
Systemic lupus erythematosus
Intestinal adhesions
Sugar-induced hypomotility
Radiation damage

Low secretory IgA

Weak ileocecal valve

Decreased motility (peristalsis) in the small intestine due to a motility disorder (e.g., systemic sclerosis) or a meal high in refined sugar can contribute to small intestinal bacterial overgrowth.[16,17] A low immune function, food allergies, stress, and other factors associated with a reduced level of secretory IgA—the antibody that protects and lines mucous membranes—can also contribute to bacterial overgrowth in the small intestine. And finally, a weak ileocecal valve (the valve that separates the bacteria-rich colon contents from the ileum, the final segment of the small intestine) can lead to overpopulation of the small intestinal tract with bacteria. A weak ileocecal valve is most often the consequence of long-term constipation or straining excessively at defecation. In both of these cases a low-fiber diet is most often responsible.

Treating Small Intestinal Bacterial Overgrowth

Obviously, addressing the cause of the small intestinal bacterial overgrowth is the first step. The subject of decreased digestive secretions is handled in Chapter 2. As for decreased motility, this most often is a result of a meal that is too high in sugar.[17] The mechanism is simple. When blood sugar levels rise too rapidly, a signal is sent to the gastrointestinal tract to slow down. Since glucose is primarily absorbed in the duodenum and jejunum, the message affects this portion of the gastrointestinal tract the most. The result is that the duodenum and jejunum become *atonic*—meaning that they literally stop functioning in the propulsion of chyme through the intestinal tract via peristalsis.

Restoring secretory IgA levels to normal involves eliminating food allergies (see Chapter 6) and enhancing immune function. Stress is particularly detrimental to secretory IgA. This effect offers an additional explanation as to why stressful events tend to worsen gastrointestinal function and food allergies. How to deal with stress more effectively is discussed on page 78 in "Stress and the Irritable Bowel Syndrome."

Clinically, I have found pancreatic enzymes and goldenseal root extract to provide a good answer to small intestinal bacterial overgrowth. Goldenseal is also discussed more fully on page 90 in Chapter 5. In addition to exerting broad-spectrum antibiotic activity (including activity against the yeast *Candida albicans*), the chief component of goldenseal, berberine, has been shown to inhibit the bacterial enzyme (decarboxylase) that converts the amino acids into vasoactive amines.[18] Because the protein-digesting enzymes from the pancreas are largely responsible for keeping the small intestine free from bacteria as well as parasites (yeast, protozoa, and intestinal worms)[15], a lack of proteases or other digestive secretions greatly increases an individual's risk of getting an intestinal infection, including chronic candida infections of the gastrointestinal tract. Follow the dosage recommendations given for goldenseal on page 94 and pancreatic enzymes on page 31.

Candidiasis

An overgrowth in the gastrointestinal tract of the usually benign yeast *Candida albicans* is now becoming recognized as a complex syndrome known as the *yeast syndrome* or *chronic candidiasis*. The overgrowth of candida is believed to cause a wide variety of symptoms in virtually every system of the body, with the gastrointestinal, genitourinary, endocrine, nervous, and immune systems being the most susceptible. Eventually this syndrome will likely be replaced by a more comprehensive term to include small intestinal bacterial overgrowth.

Although chronic candidiasis has been clinically defined for a long time, it was not until Orion Truss published *The Missing Diagnosis* (P.O. Box 26508, Birmingham, AL, 1983) and William Crook published *The Yeast Connection* (Professional Books, Jackson, TN, 1984) that the public and many physicians became aware of the magnitude of the problem.

The diagnosis of chronic candidiasis is often quite difficult because there is no single specific diagnostic test. Stool cultures and elevated antibody levels due to candida are useful diagnostic aids, but they should not be relied upon for diagnosis. The best method for diagnosing chronic candidiasis is a detailed medical history and patient questionnaire. The candida questionnaire that I use is on page 54.

Candida Questionnaire

	Point Score

History

1. Have you taken tetracycline or other antibiotics for acne for one month or longer? — 25

2. Have you, at any time in your life, taken other broad-spectrum antibiotics for respiratory, urinary, or other infections for two months or longer, or in short courses four or more times in a one-year period? — 20

3. Have you ever taken a broad-spectrum antibiotic (even a single course)? — 6

4. Have you, at any time in your life, been bothered by persistent prostatitis, vaginitis, or other problems affecting your reproductive organs? — 25

5. Have you been pregnant . . .

   One time? — 3

   Two or more times? — 5

6. Have you taken birth control pills . . .

   For six months to two years? — 8

   For more than two years? — 15

7. Have you taken prednisone or other cortisone-type drugs . . .

   For two weeks or less? — 6

   For more than two weeks? — 15

8. Does exposure to perfumes, insecticides, fabric shop odors, and other chemicals provoke . . .

   Mild symptoms? — 5

   Moderate to severe symptoms? — 20

9. Are your symptoms worse on damp, muggy days or in moldy places? — 20

10. Have you had athlete's foot, ringworm, "jock itch," or other chronic infections of the skin or nails?

    Mild to moderate? — 10

    Severe or persistent? — 20

11. Do you crave sugar? — 10

12. Do you crave breads? — 10

Candida Questionnaire *(continued)*

13. Do you crave alcoholic beverages?	10
14. Does tobacco smoke *really* bother you?	10
Total Score of This Section	_____

Major Symptoms

For each of your symptoms, enter the appropriate figure in the Point Score column.

Score column:

> If a symptom is occasional or mild, score 3 points
> If a symptom is frequent and/or moderately severe, score 6 points
> If a symptom is severe and/or disabling, score 9 points

POINT SCORE

1. Fatigue or lethargy _____
2. Feeling of being "drained" _____
3. Poor memory _____
4. Feeling "spacey" or "unreal" _____
5. Depression _____
6. Numbness, burning, or tingling _____
7. Muscle aches _____
8. Muscle weakness or paralysis _____
9. Pain and/or swelling in joints _____
10. Abdominal pain _____
11. Constipation _____
12. Diarrhea _____
13. Bloating _____
14. Persistent vaginal itch _____
15. Persistent vaginal burning _____
16. Prostatitis _____
17. Impotence _____
18. Loss of sexual desire _____
19. Endometriosis _____
20. Cramps and/or other menstrual irregularities _____
21. Premenstrual tension _____

Continued

Candida Questionnaire *(continued)*

22. Spots in front of eyes   _____
23. Erratic vision   _____

Total Score of This Section   _____

Other Symptoms

For each of your symptoms, enter the appropriate figure in the Point Score column.

Score column:

If a symptom is occasional or mild, score 1 point
If a symptom is frequent and/or moderately severe,
    score 2 points
If a symptom is severe and/or disabling, score 3 points

POINT SCORE

1. Drowsiness   _____
2. Irritability   _____
3. Incoordination   _____
4. Inability to concentrate   _____
5. Frequent mood swings   _____
6. Headache   _____
7. Dizziness/loss of balance   _____
8. Pressure above ears, feeling of head
   swelling and tingling   _____
9. Itching   _____
10. Other rashes   _____
11. Heartburn   _____
12. Indigestion   _____
13. Belching and intestinal gas   _____
14. Mucus in stools   _____
15. Hemorrhoids   _____
16. Dry mouth   _____
17. Rash or blisters in mouth   _____
18. Bad breath   _____
19. Joint swelling or arthritis   _____
20. Nasal congestion or discharge   _____
21. Postnasal drip   _____

Candida Questionnaire *(continued)*

22. Nasal itching _____
23. Sore or dry throat _____
24. Cough _____
25. Pain or tightness in chest _____
26. Wheezing or shortness of breath _____
27. Urinary urgency or frequency _____
28. Burning on urination _____
29. Failing vision _____
30. Burning or tearing of eyes _____
31. Recurrent infections or fluid in ears _____
32. Ear pain or deafness _____

Total Score of This Section _____

Total Score of All Three Sections _____

Interpretation

	Women	Men
Yeast-connected health problems are almost certainly present	>180	>140
Yeast-connected health problems are probably present	120–180	90–140
Yeast-connected health problems are possibly present	60–119	40–89
Yeast-connected health problems are less likely present	<60	<40

Adapted from Crook, W. G., *The Yeast Connection,* 2nd ed., Professional Books, Jackson, TN, 1984.

Getting Rid of Candida

Getting rid of candida involves an approach similar to that given above for small intestinal bacterial overgrowth. In particular, hydrochloric acid, pancreatic enzymes, and bile are potent natural factors that inhibit the overgrowth of candida. Promoting improved digestion with the aid of hydrochloric acid and pancreatic enzyme preparations, as detailed in Chapter 2, is extremely important in relieving chronic candidiasis. The difference in treating candidiasis compared to small intestinal bacterial overgrowth is that in chronic candidiasis the yeast becomes more firmly entrenched in the lining of the intestinal tract and the colon serves as a reservoir for the yeast. Therefore, a more aggressive approach is warranted.

A Comprehensive Approach to Treatment

Simply trying to kill the candida with a drug is like trying to weed your garden by simply cutting the weed instead of pulling it out by the roots. Drugs like nystatin, ketoconazol, and diflucan rarely produce significant long-term results because they fail to address the underlying factors that promote candida overgrowth.

In order to get to the root of the candida problem, a comprehensive approach is necessary. I realize that my recommendations may seem to be a bit overwhelming for this condition, but I urge you to employ all of them if you want to really get rid of this problem.

Diet is the first step. Avoid those foods that promote candida growth including high-sugar foods, alcohol, foods with a high content of yeast or mold (cheeses, dried fruits, and peanuts), and milk and milk products. In addition, it is important to avoid food allergies (discussed in Chapter 6).

Improving Liver Function in Chronic Candidiasis

Candida patients usually exhibit multiple chemical sensitivities and allergies, an indicator that detoxification reactions are stressed. Therefore, the candida patient needs to support liver function. In fact, improving the health of the liver may be one of the most critical factors in the successful treatment of candidiasis. In animal experiments, damaging the liver led to candida overgrowth.[19]

Candida patients should take extra choline, methionine, betaine, and folic acid to support liver function. These nutrients are often referred to as *lipotropic agents* because they promote the flow of fat and bile to and from the liver. In essence, they produce a decongestive effect on the liver and promote improved liver function and fat metabolism. Most major manufacturers of nutritional supplements offer lipotropic formulas. When taking a lipotropic formula, the most important thing is to take enough of the formula to provide a daily dose of 1,000 mg of choline and 500 mg of methionine and/or cysteine.

Enhancing Immune Function

Another crucial loop in our defensive chain against candida overgrowth is enhancing the immune system. This may simply involve taking a high potency multiple vitamin-mineral formula (follow the guidelines given on page 167 in Chapter 8) and following the recommendations for dealing with stress more effectively given on page 79 in Chapter 5. In most cases, however, in addition to these measures I recommend promoting optimal thymus gland activity by (1) preventing thymic involution or shrinkage by ensuring adequate dietary intake of antioxidant nutrients such as carotenes, vitamin C, vitamin E, zinc, and selenium; (2) supplying nutrients that are required in the manufacture or action of thymic hormones; and (3) using products containing concentrates of calf thymus tissue.

The thymus gland is the main organ of the immune system and to a very large extent, the health of the thymus determines the health of the immune system. The thymus is responsible for many immune system functions including the production of T lymphocytes, a type of white blood cell responsible for *cell-mediated immunity*. Cell-mediated immunity refers to immune mechanisms not controlled or mediated by antibodies. Cell-mediated immunity is extremely important in the body's resistance to infection by yeast (including candida), fungi, mold-like bacteria, parasites, and viruses (including Herpes simplex, Epstein-Barr, and viruses that cause hepatitis). If an individual is suffering from an infection of these organisms, it is a good indication that their cell-mediated immunity is not functioning up to par. Cell-mediated immunity is also critical in protecting against the development of cancer, auto-immune disorders like rheumatoid arthritis, and allergies.

Antioxidants and Thymus Function   The thymus gland shows maximum development immediately after birth. During the aging process, the thymus gland undergoes a process of shrinkage or involution. The reason for this involution is that the thymus gland is extremely susceptible to free radical and oxidative damage caused by stress, radiation, infection, and chronic illness. It is very important to supplement the diet with antioxidants such as vitamin C, vitamin E, selenium, and zinc. All of these nutrients have been shown to prevent thymic involution and enhance cell-mediated immune functions. (Follow the recommendations given on page 167 in Chapter 8.)

Nutrients Required for Thymic Hormone Manufacture or Action   Many nutrients function as important cofactors in the manufacture, secretion, and function of thymic hormones. A deficiency of any one of these nutrients results in decreased thymic hormone action and impaired immune function. Zinc, vitamin B_6, and vitamin C are perhaps the most critical nutrients. Supplementation with these nutrients has been shown to increase thymic hormone function and cell-mediated immunity. Again, following the guidelines given on page 167 in Chapter 8 will provide optimal levels of these important nutrients.

Enhancing Thymus Function with Thymus Extracts A substantial amount of clinical data supports the effectiveness of orally administered calf thymus extracts in restoring and enhancing immune function.[20,21] The effectiveness of thymus extract is reflective of broad-spectrum immune system enhancement presumably mediated by improved thymus gland activity. This effect fits in nicely with one of the basic concepts of glandular therapy, i.e., that the oral ingestion of glandular material of a certain animal gland will strengthen the corresponding human gland. The result is a broad general effect indicative of improved glandular function.

Because there are no quality control procedures or standards enforced in the glandular industry, the correct dosage of thymus extract will vary from one manufacturer to another.

From a practical view, products concentrated and standardized for polypeptide content are preferable to crude preparations. Based on current clinical research, the daily dose should be equivalent to 120 mg of pure polypeptides, with molecular weights less than 10,000 or roughly 500 mg of the crude polypeptide fraction. No side effects or adverse effects have been reported with the use of thymus preparations.

Killing Candida

The next step in treating candidiasis is using any of a number of nutritional and herbal substances that are designed to kill off the organism. Pancreatic enzymes and goldenseal root are helpful (see pages 31 and 90). Caprylic acid and garlic preparations have been used for many years by alternative health care professionals in the treatment of candida overgrowth. Garlic has been shown to be more potent than nystatin, gentian violet, and many other anti-candida agents in experimental studies.[22,23] Garlic preparations producing a high allicin-potential may offer the greatest benefit. Consider using commercial preparations concentrated for alliin because alliin is relatively odorless until it is converted to allicin in the body. For best results, products standardized for alliin content are preferred. The dosage should provide a daily dose of 8 mg alliin.

Caprylic acid (a naturally occurring short-chain fatty acid that is made from coconut oil) has also demonstrated good anti-candida effects. However, because caprylic acid is readily absorbed in the intestines, it is necessary to take timed-released or enteric-coated caprylic acid formulas to allow for gradual release throughout the entire intestinal tract.[24]

Recently, many alternative health care physicians have begun using stronger natural anti-candida agents such as grapefruit seed extract or specially prepared volatile oil preparations from peppermint, thyme, and oregano. According to the many physicians who are using these "new wave" natural anti-candida formulas, they are more effective than caprylic acid and garlic products. The volatile oil products are especially promising because they have demonstrated significant activity against *Candida albicans* and have been shown to be more potent than caprylic acid.

A recent study compared the anti-candida effect of oregano oil to caprylic acid.[25] The results of the study indicated that the anti-candida activity of oregano oil is at least 100 times more potent than caprylic acid. Since the volatile oils are quickly absorbed as well as associated with inducing heartburn, an enteric-coating is recommended to ensure delivery to the small and large intestine.

An effective dosage for an enteric-coated volatile oil preparation is 0.2 to 0.4 ml twice daily between meals.

Lactobacillus Inhibits Candida

Although the health-promoting effects of the bacteria *Lactobacillus acidophilus* are discussed more fully in Chapter 5 beginning on page 81, in short, *L. acidophilus* has been shown to retard the growth of candida in culture media and is thought to be one of the natural protective measures against candida overgrowth.[26] The appropriate dosage of a commercial *L. acidophilus* supplement is based upon the number of live organisms. The ingestion of 5 to 10 billion viable *L. acidophilus* or *B. bifidum* cells daily is a sufficient dosage for most people with chronic candidiasis. Amounts exceeding this may induce mild gastrointestinal disturbances, while smaller amounts may not be able to colonize the gastrointestinal tract.

Treating Chronic Candidiasis: A Summary of Steps

1. Eliminate the use of antibiotics, steroids, immune-suppressing drugs, and birth control pills (unless there is absolute medical necessity).

2. Follow these special dietary guidelines:

   Do not eat foods high in sugar.

   Do not eat foods with a high content of yeast or mold including alcoholic beverages, cheeses, dried fruits, melons, and peanuts.

   Do not eat milk and milk products due to their high content of lactose (milk sugar) and trace levels of antibiotics.

   Avoid all known or suspected food allergies (see Chapter 6).

3. Improve liver function by taking a lipotropic formula.

4. Take a high potency multiple vitamin-mineral formula.

5. Enhance immune function if necessary.

6. Ingest 5 to 10 billion viable *L. acidophilus* or *B. bifidum* cells daily.

7. Use nutritional and/or herbal supplements, such as enteric-coated volatile oil preparations, probiotics, and caprylic acid, that help control against yeast overgrowth and promote a healthy bacterial flora.

8. Promote the elimination of candida toxins by taking 5 grams of a water-soluble fiber source such as guar gum, psyllium seed, or pectin, which can bind to toxins in the gut and promote their excretion, at night before retiring.

The Leaky Gut

While the concept of the leaky gut (increased gastro-intestinal permeability) is also discussed in the context of increased colon permeability and food allergy (see Chapters 5 and 6), it is introduced here because it also may be the result of celiac disease, small intestinal bacterial over-growth, and chronic candidiasis. Increased gastrointestinal permeability leads to absorption of large food particles, bacterial components, and various toxic chemicals. Depending upon the nature of the permeating molecules, and the physiological state of the host, symptoms may be similar to those described for chronic candidiasis. Some of the most damaging molecules are yeast and bacterial components such as endotoxins (cellular membranes of gram-negative bacteria) and antigenic material (substances that cause the immune system to form antibodies against it).

Absorption of these compounds is linked to a growing list of health conditions, many of which are a result of the body's immune-system response to the endotoxin or antigen.[27-30] Examples of conditions linked to increased absorption of bacterial components include arthritis (both rheumatoid and osteoarthritis); autoimmune diseases such as Hashimoto's thyroiditis, scleroderma, systemic lupus erythematosus, and ankylosing spondylitis; cirrhosis of the liver (alcohol increases gut permeability); acne; psoriasis; and pancreatitis. In addition, increased gut permeability due to chronic inflammation is a hallmark feature of over 100 disorders, known as extra-intestinal lesions (EIL), which constitute a diverse group of systemic complications of Crohn's disease and ulcerative colitis (described in Chapter 8).[31]

Diagnosis of a leaky gut is fairly straightforward. It involves the administration of two sugars—mannitol and lactulose. Mannitol is a small sugar molecule that is quickly taken up by intestinal cells and transported into the system. Lactulose, on the other hand, is a larger molecule that should not be taken up by intestinal cells. However, if the junction between the cells is not tight (i.e., if it is leaky), lactulose will be absorbed. Therefore, mannitol serves as a marker for general absorption and lactulose serves as an indicator of increased intestinal permeability. Since neither sugar is metabolized, a six-hour urine measurement after administration of mannitol and lactulose according to standard guidelines can detect a leaky gut.

Normally, the percentage of mannitol that is recovered is between 5% to 25% and the percentage of lactulose that is recovered is 0.1% to 0.8%. If the levels of lactulose and mannitol are both higher, this indicates general increased intestinal permeability. If the levels of mannitol and lactulose are both decreased, this reflects malabsorption. And if the level of lactulose is increased and the level of mannitol is decreased or the ratio of lactulose to mannitol is increased, this may indicate damage to absorptive surfaces similar to the damage associated with celiac disease.

In most circumstances, correcting the leaky gut requires addressing the factors that can lead to inflammation—e.g.,

Crohn's disease (Chapter 8), celiac disease (discussed on page 46), and food allergies (Chapter 6), bacterial overgrowth in the small intestine, and the overgrowth of candida.

Final Comments

Because the small intestine is the primary site where the digestive and assimilative processes occur, there is a great deal going on in this organ. Altered small intestine function and integrity have significant repercussions on nutritional status and overall health. Proper small intestine function requires effective digestive secretions coupled with a fully functional absorptive surface and barrier. Conditions discussed in this chapter are best treated by addressing the underlying issues such as food intolerance/allergy, lack of digestive secretions, low immune status, and too much sugar in the diet.

5

Colon Disorders

The large intestine is really not involved in digestion to any significant extent although it does function in the absorption of water and electrolytes (salts). Its primary function is to provide temporary storage for waste products and the formation of stool. The health of the colon is largely determined by the amount of dietary fiber a person consumes. Without enough dietary fiber, waste material tends to accumulate. Equally as important as proper digestion is the proper elimination of waste products.

This chapter will discuss several conditions that affect the colon, including constipation, diverticular disease, hemorrhoids, irritable bowel syndrome, dysbiosis, and parasitic infections.

Constipation

Constipation affects over 4 million people in the United States on a regular basis.[1] This high rate of constipation

Table 5.1   Causes of Constipation

Dietary	Highly refined and low-fiber foods, inadequate fluid intake
Physical inactivity	Inadequate exercise, prolonged bed rest
Pregnancy	
Advanced age	
Drugs	Anesthetics, antacids (aluminum and calcium salts), anticholinergics (bethanechol, carbachol, pilocarpine, physostigmine, ambenonium), anticonvulsants, antidepressants (tricyclics, monoamine oxidase inhibitors), antihypertensives, anti-parkinsonism drugs, antipsychotics (phenothiazines), beta-adrenergic blocking agents (propanolol), bismuth salts, diuretics, iron salts, laxatives and cathartics (chronic use), muscle relaxants, opiates, toxic metals (arsenic, lead, mercury)
Metabolic abnormalities	Low potassium stores, diabetes, kidney disease
Endocrine abnormalities	Low thyroid function, elevated calcium levels, pituitary disorders
Structural abnormalities	Abnormalities in the structure or anatomy of the bowel
Bowel diseases	Diverticulosis, irritable bowel syndrome (alternating diarrhea and constipation), tumors
Neurogenic abnormalities	Nerve disorders of the bowel (aganglionosis, autonomic neuropathy), spinal cord disorders (trauma, multiple sclerosis, tabes dorsalis), disorders of the splanchnic nerves (tumors, trauma), cerebral disorders (strokes, parkinsonism, neoplasm)
Enemas	chronic use

translates to over $400 million in annual sales of laxatives in the United States. There are a number of possible causes of constipation (see Table 5.1), but the most common cause of constipation is simply a low-fiber diet.

Relieving Constipation

Constipation will usually respond to a high-fiber diet, plentiful fluid consumption, and exercise. Unfortunately, instead of following this natural approach, many people have become dependent upon laxatives.

Increasing dietary fiber is an effective treatment of chronic constipation. High levels of dietary fiber increase both the frequency and quantity of bowel movements, decrease the transit time of stools, decrease the absorption of toxins from the stool, and appear to be a preventive factor in several diseases. Particularly effective in relieving constipation are bran and prunes. The typical recommendation for bran is ½ cup of bran cereal, increasing to 1½ cups over several weeks. Whole prunes as well as prune juice possess good laxative effects. Eight ounces of juice (or four to six prunes) is usually an effective dose.

Be sure that you are consuming enough liquids. Drink at least six to eight glasses of water per day. In addition, try to consume 25 to 35 grams of fiber each day from the foods listed in Table 5.2.

If you need additional support, consider using fiber-formula laxatives. These formulas act as bulking agents. They can be composed of natural plant fibers derived from psyllium seed, kelp, agar, pectin, and plant gums such as karaya and guar. Or they can be purified semi-synthetic polysaccharides such as methyl-cellulose and carboxymethyl cellulose sodium. Psyllium-containing laxatives are the most popular and usually the most effective. Fiber formulas are the laxatives that most closely approximate the natural mechanism which promotes a bowel movement.

Retraining Your Bowels

If you have been using stimulant laxatives, even natural ones such as Cascara sagrada (*Rhamnus purshiana*) or

Table 5.2   Dietary Fiber Content of Selected Foods

Food	Serving	Calories	Grams of fiber
Fruits (no more than 4 servings daily)			
Apple (with skin)	1 medium	81	3.5
Banana	1 medium	105	2.4
Cantaloupe	¼ melon	30	1.0
Cherries, sweet	10	49	1.2
Grapefruit	½ medium	38	1.6
Orange	1 medium	62	2.6
Peach (with skin)	1	37	1.9
Pear (with skin)	½ large	61	3.1
Prunes	3	60	3.0
Raisins	¼ cup	106	3.1
Raspberries	½ cup	35	3.1
Strawberries	1 cup	45	3.0
Vegetables, Raw (as many servings as desired)			
Bean sprouts	½ cup	13	1.5
Celery, diced	½ cup	10	1.1
Cucumber	½ cup	8	0.4
Lettuce	1 cup	10	0.9
Mushrooms	½ cup	10	1.5
Pepper, green	½ cup	9	0.5
Spinach	1 cup	8	1.2
Tomato	1 medium	20	1.5
Vegetables, Cooked (as many servings as desired)			
Asparagus, cut	1 cup	30	2.0
Beans, green	1 cup	32	3.2
Broccoli	1 cup	40	4.4
Brussels sprouts	1 cup	56	4.6
Cabbage	1 cup	30	2.8
Carrots	1 cup	48	4.6
Cauliflower	1 cup	28	2.2
Corn	½ cup	87	2.9
Kale	1 cup	44	2.8
Parsnip	1 cup	102	5.4

Table 5.2 Dietary Fiber Content of Selected Foods *(continued)*

Food	Serving	Calories	Grams of fiber
Potato (with skin)	1 medium	106	2.5
Potato (without skin)	1 medium	97	1.4
Spinach	1 cup	42	4.2
Sweet potatoes	1 medium	160	3.4
Zucchini	1 cup	22	3.6
Legumes			
Baked beans	½ cup	155	8.8
Dried peas, cooked	½ cup	115	4.7
Kidney beans, cooked	½ cup	110	7.3
Lima beans, cooked	½ cup	64	4.5
Lentils, cooked	½ cup	97	3.7
Navy beans, cooked	½ cup	112	6.0
Breakfast cereals (no more than 2 servings daily)			
All-Bran	⅓ cup	71	8.5
Bran Chex	⅔ cup	91	4.6
Corn Bran	⅔ cup	98	5.4
Oatmeal	¾ cup	108	1.6
Raisin Bran	⅔ cup	115	4.0
Shredded Wheat	⅔ cup	102	2.6

senna (*Cassia senna*), you will need to "retrain" your bowels. Listed below are the recommended rules for reestablishing bowel regularity as presented in the *Encyclopedia of Natural Medicine* (Murray, M. T. and Pizzorno, J. E., Prima Publishing, 1991). The recommended procedure will take four to six weeks.

1. Find and eliminate known causes of constipation.
2. Never repress an urge to defecate.
3. Eat a high-fiber diet, particularly fruits and vegetables.

4. Drink six to eight glasses of water per day.
5. Sit on the toilet at the same time every day (even when the urge to defecate is not present), preferably immediately after breakfast or exercise.
6. Exercise for at least 20 minutes, three times per week.
7. Stop using laxatives (except as discussed below to reestablish bowel activity) and enemas.

> Week one: Every night before bed take a stimulant laxative containing either cascara or senna. Take the lowest amount necessary to reliably ensure a bowel movement every morning.

> Weekly thereafter: Each week decrease dosage by half. If constipation recurs, go back to the previous week's dosage. Decrease dosage if diarrhea occurs.

Diverticular Disease

Diverticula are small sacs caused by the protrusion of the inner lining of the colon into areas of weakness in the colon wall. The term *diverticulosis* signifies the presence of diverticula in the colon. Most often the presence of diverticula is without symptom, however, if the diverticula becomes inflamed, perforated, or impacted it is referred to as *diverticulitis*. Only about 20% of people with diverticulosis develop diverticulitis. Symptoms of diverticulitis include episodes of lower abdominal pain and cramping, changes in bowel habits (constipation or diarrhea), and a sense of fullness in the abdomen. In more severe cases, fever may be present along with tenderness and rigidity of the abdomen over the area of the intestine involved.

Treatment of diverticular disease involves the consumption of a high-fiber diet. In severe cases of diverticulitis, an antibiotic may be warranted. If you are having symptoms suggestive of diverticulitis, consult a physician immediately. For mild cases, I would recommend goldenseal root. Follow the recommendations given on page 94.

Hemorrhoids

Hemorrhoids are basically varicose veins of the rectum. They may be near the beginning of the anal canal (internal hemorrhoids) or at the anal opening (external hemorrhoids). Hemorrhoids are extremely common in the United States, as well as other industrialized countries. Estimates have indicated that 50% of persons over 50 years of age have symptomatic hemorrhoidal disease and up to one-third of the total U.S. population has hemorrhoids to some degree.

Because the venous system supplying the rectal area contains no valves, factors that increase venous congestion in the region can precipitate hemorrhoid formation. These factors include increasing intra-abdominal pressure (e.g., defecation, pregnancy, coughing, sneezing, vomiting, physical exertion, and portal hypertension due to cirrhosis), a low-fiber diet-induced increase in straining during defecation, and standing or sitting for prolonged periods of time.

The symptoms most often associated with hemorrhoids include burning, pain, inflammation, irritation, swelling, bleeding, and seepage. Itching is rarely directly due to hemorrhoids except when there is mucus discharge from prolapsing internal hemorrhoids. The most common causes of anal itching include tissue trauma due to excessive use of harsh toilet paper, *Candida albicans,* parasitic infections, and allergies.

Increase Fiber to Treat and Prevent Hemorrhoids

In contrast to the United States, hemorrhoids are rarely seen in parts of the world where high-fiber, unrefined diets are consumed.[1] A low-fiber diet, high in refined foods, contributes greatly to the development of hemorrhoids.

Individuals consuming a low-fiber diet tend to strain more during bowel movements, since their smaller and harder stools are more difficult to pass. This straining increases the pressure in the abdomen, which obstructs venous return. The increased pressure increases pelvic congestion and may significantly weaken the veins, causing hemorrhoids to form.

A high-fiber diet is perhaps the most important component in the prevention of hemorrhoids. A diet rich in vegetables, fruits, legumes, and whole grains promotes peristalsis, and many fiber components attract water and form a gelatinous mass that keeps the stools soft, bulky, and easy to pass. The net effect of a high-fiber diet is significantly less straining during defecation. Natural bulking agents, particularly powdered psyllium seed husks, can also be used to reduce fecal straining and relieve hemorrhoids.[2] Take 3 to 5 grams of psyllium fiber per day.

Other Treatments for Hemorrhoids

A warm sitz bath is an effective noninvasive treatment for uncomplicated hemorrhoids. A sitz bath is a partial immersion bath of the pelvic region. The temperature of the water in the warm sitz bath should be between 100 to 105 degrees Fahrenheit.

The use of medicated creams, pads, suppositories, and ointments can provide some temporary relief. Many over-the-counter products, as well as products in health food stores for hemorrhoids, contain natural ingredients such as witch hazel (*Hamamelis* water), shark liver oil, cod liver oil, cocoa butter, Peruvian balsam, vitamin E, zinc oxide, live yeast cell derivative, and allantoin. Use these products according to the directions on the label.

To strengthen the blood vessels, consume the key nutrients vitamin C (500 to 1,500 mg) and zinc (15 to 30 mg) daily; citrus bioflavonoids or a special aortic extract may also prove useful. Citrus bioflavonoids (specifically, hydroxy-ethyl-rutosides) have been shown to be effective in the treatment of hemorrhoids, including hemorrhoids due to pregnancy.[2,3] An effective dosage would be 3,000 to 6,000 mg daily. Even more effective is a special extract of bovine (beef) aortic glycosaminogly-cans (GAGs). Over 50 clinical studies have shown that an orally administered complex of aortic GAGs is effective in treating a number of vascular disorders including hemorrhoids, cerebral and peripheral arterial insuffi-ciency, venous insufficiency and varicose veins, vascular retinopathies including macular degeneration, and post-surgical edema. In head-to-head comparison studies with bioflavonoids, the aortic extract produced far better re-sults in relieving hemorrhoids. In fact, the authors of the study suggested that it should be used as the "drug of first choice" in the nonsurgical treatment of acute hemor-rhoidal pain and disease.[4] The standard dosage is 50 mg, twice daily.

Irritable Bowel Syndrome

Irritable bowel syndrome (IBS) is a very common condi-tion in which the large intestine (colon) fails to function properly. Estimates suggest that approximately 15% of the U.S. population has suffered from IBS.

IBS is also known as nervous indigestion, spastic colitis, mucous colitis, and intestinal neurosis. Characteristic symptoms of IBS can include a combination of any of the following: abdominal pain and distension; more frequent bowel movements with pain; relief of pain with bowel movements; constipation; diarrhea; excessive production of mucus in the colon; symptoms of indigestion such as flatulence, nausea, or anorexia; and varying degrees of anxiety or depression.

Relieving the Irritable Bowel Syndrome

The irritable bowel syndrome is usually caused by either a lack of dietary fiber in the diet or food allergies or both. Simply increasing the intake of plant food in the diet is effective is most cases. What many people don't realize is that the term *dietary fiber* means the indigestible compounds in plant foods. All plant foods contain fiber, not just whole grains or bran. In fact, you may be surprised to learn that one pear or one serving of broccoli contains more fiber than four slices of whole grain bread. You would have to eat 10 slices of whole grain bread to equal the amount of fiber in a cup of cooked navy beans!

Not only is there more fiber in many other plant foods than in whole grains, but it is a better type of fiber. The fiber in vegetables, fruits, oat bran, and legumes (beans, peas, etc.) is largely water soluble rather than the insoluble fiber of wheat bran. This is important because the water-soluble fibers produce a softer and gentler stool, which is easier to pass than the insoluble fibers. They also lower cholesterol levels.

In addition to eating more high-fiber foods, you may want to use a fiber formula rich in water-soluble fibers. Choose formulas that contain one or more of these fiber sources: psyllium seed husks, pectin, oat bran, guar gum, beet fiber, carrot fiber. For best results, I recommend that you take enough of the formula to provide 3 to 5 grams of fiber at night an hour or so before going to bed.

While you want to increase your intake of dietary fiber, there is one thing you absolutely must avoid—white table sugar (sucrose). Sugar has a very detrimental effect on bowel function, particularly in patients with IBS.[5]

Food allergies are also a frequent cause of IBS; the majority of patients with IBS (approximately two-thirds) have at least one food allergy, and some have multiple food allergies.[6,7] Many IBS patients have other symptoms suggestive of food allergy, such as heart palpitation, hyperventilation, fatigue, excessive sweating, and headaches.

If you have increased your intake of dietary fiber, quit eating sugar, and eliminated food allergies yet still have symptoms of IBS, you may want to try drinking some peppermint tea. Or, better yet, use peppermint oil provided in enteric-coated preparations, which prevent the oil from being released in the stomach. Without enteric coating, peppermint oil tends to produce heartburn. With the coating, the peppermint oil travels to the small and large intestines where it relaxes intestinal muscles. Several clinical studies have demonstrated that enteric-coated peppermint oil is quite effective in reducing the abdominal symptoms of the irritable bowel syndrome.[8,9]

One of the central findings in IBS is a hypercontractility (excessive contraction) of intestinal smooth muscle. Peppermint oil inhibits the hypercontractility of intestinal smooth muscle, making it useful in cases of IBS as well as intestinal colic (it can be used safely in children over four years of age).

In addition to reducing hypercontractility, peppermint oil may also work by destroying the yeast *Candida albicans* (discussed on page 53). The typical dosage is 0.2 to 0.4 ml twice daily between meals.

Stress and the Irritable Bowel Syndrome

Almost all patients with IBS complain of mental/emotional problems such as anxiety, fatigue, hostile feelings, depression, and sleep disturbances.[10] There are several theories that link psychological factors to the symptoms of IBS.[11] The "learning model" maintains that when exposed to stressful situations some children learn to develop gastrointestinal symptoms to cope with the stress. Another theory holds that IBS is a manifestation of depression or chronic anxiety or both. Personality assessments of IBS sufferers have shown them to have higher than average anxiety levels and a greater feeling of depression.[12] However, these studies were based on personality assessments after the individuals developed IBS. It has since been determined by pre-illness personality assessment that IBS sufferers have normal personality profiles before their illness. Therefore, many of the common psychological symptoms of IBS sufferers may be either a result of the bowel disturbances or be caused by a problem such as stress, food allergy, environmental illness, or candidiasis.

Some researchers believe that IBS sufferers have difficulty in adapting to life events, although this theory has not been fully demonstrated in clinical studies. However, increased contractions of the colon during exposure to stressful situations has been shown to occur in both normal subjects and those suffering IBS.[13] This could account for the increased abdominal pain and irregular bowel functions experienced by most people during periods of emotional stress.

Various methods have been used to tackle these psychological factors as a part of the standard medical treatment of IBS. Psychotherapy in the form of biofeedback or short-term individual counseling has sometimes proved successful.[14,15] An increase in physical exercise also appears to be helpful for IBS patients suffering from stress.

Many people find that daily leisurely walks markedly reduce their symptoms, probably due to the known stress-reduction effects of exercise.

Stress and Digestion

During the stress response, the sympathetic arm of the autonomic nervous system dominates the parasympathetic. While the sympathetic nervous system stimulates the fight-or-flight response, it is the parasympathetic that is responsible for the process of digestion, repair, restoration, and rejuvenation. If a person is in a stressed state, the body is programmed to shunt blood and energy away from the digestive tract in favor of the skeletal muscles and brain (if a lion is chasing you, for example, it is better to direct blood and energy to these areas).

Regularly achieving a relaxed state (i.e., learning to calm the mind and body) is extremely important in relieving stress as well as improving digestion. The *relaxation response* is a term that was coined by Harvard professor and cardiologist Herbert Benson, M.D., in the early 1970s to describe a physiological response that is just the opposite of the stress response. With the relaxation response, the parasympathetic nervous system dominates. To achieve the relaxation response, a variety of techniques can be used. Some of the techniques you can choose from include meditation, prayer, progressive relaxation, self-hypnosis, and biofeedback. The type of relaxation technique best for each person is totally individual. It really doesn't matter which technique you choose, as long as it produces a state of deep relaxation for you. The important thing is that at least 5 to 10 minutes be set aside each day for the performance of a relaxation technique. These sessions will trigger the parasympathetic nervous system and enhance digestion. For more information on stress reduction, consult my book on *Stress, Anxiety, and Insomnia* (Prima, 1995).

Dysbiosis

The microecology of the human is an incredibly complex ecosystem; there are at least 500 different species of microflora in the human gastrointestinal tract.[16] In fact, there are nine times as many bacteria in the gastrointestinal tract as there are cells in the human body. The type and number of gut bacteria play an important role in determining health and disease. A state of altered bacterial flora in the gut has become popularly known as *dysbiosis*. The term was first used by noted Russian scientist Elie Metchnikoff to reflect a state of living with intestinal flora that has harmful effects. He theorized that toxic compounds produced by the bacterial breakdown of food were the cause of degenerative disease.[17] A growing body of evidence is supporting and refining Metchnikoff's theory. The major causes of dysbiosis are:

Dietary disturbances
    High protein
    High sugar
    High fat
    Low fiber
    Food allergies
Lack of digestive secretions
Stress
Antibiotic/drug therapy
Decreased immune function
Malabsorption
Intestinal infection
Altered pH

Obviously, treatment begins with addressing these major causes. In addition, it is important to "re-seed" the gastrointestinal tract with probiotics. *Probiotics* (literally translated it means "for life") is a term used to signify the health-promoting effects of "friendly bacteria." The most important friendly bacteria are *Lactobacillus acidophilus* and *Bifidobacterium bifidum*.

Probiotics

Foods fermented with lactobacilli have been, and still are, of great importance to the diets of most of the world's people. Most cultures use some form of fermented food in their diet such as yogurt, cheese, miso, or tempeh. The symbiotic relationship between humankind and lactobacilli has a long history of important nutritional and therapeutic benefits for humans.

At the turn of the century, Metchnikoff believed that yogurt was the elixir of life.[17] His theory was that putrefactive bacteria in the large intestine produce toxins that invite disease and shorten life. He believed that the eating of yogurt would cause the lactobacilli to become dominant in the colon and displace the putrefactive bacteria. For years, these claims of healthful effects from fermented foods were considered unscientific folklore. More recently, however, a substantial and growing body of scientific evidence has demonstrated that lactobacilli and fermented foods do play a significant role in human health.

Humans are not born with lactobacilli in their gastrointestinal tract. Colonization of gram-positive lactobacilli begins after birth, whereupon there is a dramatic increase in their concentration. *B. bifidum* is first introduced through breast feeding to the sterile gut of the infant, and large numbers are soon observed in the feces. Later, other bacteria (including such beneficial strains as *L. casea, L. fermentum, L. salivores, L. brevis*, etc.) become established in the gut through contact with the world. (See

Table 5.3   Lactobacilli Found in the Human Intestine

L. acidophilus	*L. fermentum*
L. bifidus (Bifidobacterium bifidum)	*L. leichmannii*
L. brevis	*L. plantarum*
L. casei	*L. salivaroes*
L. cellobiosus	

Table above.) Unfortunately, other potentially toxic bacteria also eventually cultivate the colon.

Promotion of the Proper Intestinal Environment with Probiotics

Lactobacilli have long been noted for the role they play in the prevention of and defense against diseases, particularly those of the gastrointestinal tract and vagina. As part of the normal flora of the body, they inhibit the growth of other organisms through competition for nutrients, alteration of pH and oxygen tension to levels less favorable to pathogens (disease-causing organisms), prevention of attachment of pathogens by physically covering attachment sites, and production of limiting factors such as antimicrobial factors.[16,18,19]

Lactobacilli produce a variety of factors that inhibit or antagonize other bacteria. These include metabolic end products such as organic acids (lactic and acetic acid), hydrogen peroxide, and compounds known as *bacteriocins*.[19] Although some researchers have isolated substances from lactobacilli which they have labeled *antibiotics*, these are probably more accurately described as bacteriocins. Bacteriocins are defined as proteins that are produced by certain bacteria which exert a lethal effect on closely related bacteria. In general, bacteriocins have a narrower range of activity than antibiotics and are

Table 5.4   Harmful Microorganisms Inhibited by *L. acidophilus*

Bacillus subtillis	*Salmonella typhosa*
B. cerus	*S. schottmuelleri*
B. stearothermophilus	*Shigella dysenteriae*
Candida albicans	*S. paradysenteriae*
Clostridium perfringens	*Sarcina lutea*
E. coli	*Serratia marcescens*
Klebsiella pneumoniae	*Staphylococcus aureus*
Proteus vulgaris	*Streptococcus fecalis*
Pseudomonas aeruginosa	*S. lactis*
P. flourescens	*Vibrio comma*

often more lethal. In addition to these direct effects, some researchers believe the antimicrobial activity of probiotics is also due to immune system stimulation.[20]

The earliest reported therapeutic uses of *L. acidophilus* in the 1920s suggested that their proliferation was associated with a simultaneous decrease in potentially harmful coliform bacteria (see Table 5.4). This effect has since been confirmed.[21-23] However, even though positive effects were reported, it is believed that many of the earlier commercial products were less reliable than those used in later published clinical trials because of inappropriate strains and problems in production, storage, and distribution to consumers.[24] Hence, even better results than those achieved in earlier studies should be expected if using a high-quality product.

Post-Antibiotic Therapy   Acidophilus supplementation is particularly important for preventing and treating antibiotic-induced diarrhea, candida overgrowth, and urinary tract infections. *L. acidophilus* has been shown to correct the increase of gram-negative bacteria observed following the administration of broad-spectrum antibiotics or as occurs with any acute or chronic diarrhea.[16, 25-27]

Although it is commonly believed that acidophilus supplements are not effective if taken during antibiotic therapy, research actually supports the use of *L. acidophilus* during antibiotic administration.[26,27] Reductions of friendly bacteria and/or superinfection with antibiotic-resistant flora may be prevented by administering *L. acidophilus* products during antibiotic therapy. A dosage of at least 15 to 20 billion organisms is required. I would still recommend taking the probiotic supplement as far away from the antibiotic as possible (e.g., if the antibiotic is to be taken every 8 hours, then take the probiotic 4 hours after the antibiotic).

Dosage   The dosage of a commercial probiotic supplement is based upon the number of live organisms it contains. The ingestion of 1 to 10 billion viable *L. acidophilus* or *B. bifidum* cells daily is a sufficient dosage for most people. Amounts exceeding this may induce mild gastrointestinal disturbances, while smaller amounts may not be able to colonize the gastrointestinal tract. Probiotics are extremely safe and are not associated with any side effects.

Available Forms of Probiotics   In order to provide benefit, products containing *L. acidophilus* and *B. bifidum* must provide live organisms in such a manner that they survive the hostile environment of the gastrointestinal tract. Several factors, such as species, strain, adherence, growth media, and diet are involved in successful colonization. Typically, a high-quality commercial preparation will produce greater colonization than simply eating yogurt. One of the key reasons is that yogurt is usually made with *L. bulgaricus* or *Streptococcus thermophilus*. While these two bacteria are friendly and possess some health benefits, they are only transient visitors to the gastrointestinal tract and do not colonize the colon.

Proper manufacturing, packaging, and storing of the product is necessary to ensure viability, the right amount of moisture, and freedom from contamination. Lactobacilli do not respond well to freeze-drying (lyophilization), spray drying, or conventional frozen storage. Excessive temperatures during packaging or storage can dramatically reduce viability. Also, unless the product has been shown to be stable, refrigeration is necessary. Some products do not have to be refrigerated until after the bottle has been opened.

While there are a number of excellent companies providing high-quality probiotic products, it is difficult to sort through all of the manufacturers' claims of superiority and, unfortunately, some products have been shown to contain no active *L. acidophilus*. In fact, one study conducted at the University of Washington concluded: "Most of the lactobacilli-containing products currently available [1990] either do not contain the Lactobacillus species advertised and/or contain other bacteria of questionable benefit."[28]

However, I feel most confident when recommending products that have been developed by Professor Khem M. Shahani, Ph.D., of the University of Nebraska. Dr. Shahani is considered the world's foremost expert on probiotics and is the developer of the DDS-1 strain of *L. acidophilus*— often referred to as the "super-strain" because it exerts benefits far greater than that of the more than 200 other strains of *L. acidophilus*. Dr. Shahani has authored over 190 scientific studies on the role of lactobacilli in human health. He has personally endorsed several products available in health food stores.

Promoting the Growth of Friendly Bacteria

Food components that may help promote the growth of friendly bacteria include fructo-oligosaccharides (FOS) and dietary fiber. FOS is composed of short-chain poly-saccharides and is just now entering the U.S. market. However, the Japanese market for FOS exceeded $46 million in 1990 and the number of consumer products containing purified FOS reached 450 in 1991.[29]

FOS is not digested by humans. Instead it feeds the friendly bacteria. Studies have shown FOS to increase bifidobacteria and lactobacilli in humans while simultaneously reducing colonies of detrimental bacteria. Other benefits noted with FOS supplementation are increased production of beneficial short-chain fatty acids such as butyrate, improved liver function, reduction of serum cholesterol and blood pressure, and improved elimination of toxic compounds.[29,30]

The dosage recommendation for pure FOS is 2,000 to 3,000 mg daily. Natural food sources of FOS include Jerusalem artichoke, onion, asparagus, and garlic. However, the estimated average daily ingestion of FOS from food sources is estimated to be 800 mg. Thus, the supplementation of FOS may help boost FOS intake and promote the growth of friendly bacteria—especially bifidobacteria.

Parasitic Infections

Parasites are microorganisms that live off and ultimately cause damage to their hosts. What determines whether any of the 500 normal microbial inhabitants of the human digestive tract become parasitic is whether or not they are living in harmony (symbiosis). *Candida albicans* is an example of an organism that under normal circumstances lives in harmony with its host, but if candida overgrows and is out of balance with other gut microbes it can result in problems. In general, parasites cause most of their problems by interfering with digestion and/or damaging the intestinal lining, either of which can lead to diarrhea.

Table 5.5 Common Protozoa and Helminths

Protozoa	
Amoeba	Dientamoeba fragilis
Giardia	Iodamoeba butschlii
Trichomonas	Blastocystis
Cryptosporidium	Balantidium coli
	Chilomastix

Helminths
  Roundworm (Ascaris lumbricoides)
  Pinworm (Enterobius vermicularis)
  Hookworm (Necator americanus)
  Threadworm (Strongyloides stercoralis)
  Whipworm (Trichuris trichiura)
  Tapeworms (various species)

Diarrheal diseases caused by parasites still constitute the greatest single worldwide cause of illness and death. The problem is magnified in underdeveloped countries with poor sanitation, but even in the United States diarrheal diseases are the third major cause of sickness and death. Furthermore, the ease and frequency of worldwide travel and increased migration to the United States are resulting in growing numbers of parasitic infections.

Many different types of microbes can be classified as parasites, but usually when physicians are referring to parasites they are referring to organisms known as protozoa and helminths (worms) (see Table 5.5).

While the most commonly reported symptoms of parasitic infection are diarrhea and abdominal pain, these symptoms do not occur in every case. In fact, there appears to be a growing number of individuals experiencing milder-than-usual gastrointestinal symptoms and/or symptoms not traditionally considered to be linked to parasitic infections. For example, many individuals with irritable bowel syndrome, indigestion, and poor digestion may harbor parasites that cause the symptoms. In addition, parasitic infections are often an unsuspected cause of chronic illness and fatigue.

Signs and Symptoms of Parasitic Infections

Abdominal pain and cramps

Constipation

Depressed secretory IgA

Diarrhea

Fatigue

Fever

Flatulence

Food allergy

Foul-smelling stools

Gastritis

Headaches

Hives

Increased intestinal permeability

Indigestion

Irregular bowel movements

Irritable bowel syndrome

Loss of appetite

Low back pain

Malabsorption

Weight loss

Although it is becoming increasingly popular for health writers to discuss natural measures to deal with parasites, given the potentially serious consequences of parasitic infections, I feel that diagnosis and treatment is best done under a physician's supervision. If you suspect a parasite, consult a physician (preferably a nutrition-oriented N.D., M.D., D.O., or D.C.). If you have traveled outside of the United States; suffer from a disease associated with impaired immunity (e.g., AIDS or cancer); or if you are experiencing diarrhea, fever, and abdominal pain, consult a physician immediately for proper evaluation. Detection of parasites involves collecting multiple stool samples at two to four day intervals. The stool sample is analyzed by microscopy, specialized staining techniques, and fluorescent antibodies (the antibodies attach to any parasites present and give off fluorescence). Any of the laboratories I mentioned on page 6 for the comprehensive stool and digestive analysis are capable of performing satisfactory stool exams for parasites.

Treatment of Parasitic Infections

As stated previously, treatment of parasitic infections should be supervised by a physician to ensure that the therapy is effective. A number of natural compounds can be useful in helping the body get rid of parasites. However, before selecting a natural alternative to an antibiotic in parasitic infections, I try to discern what factors may have been responsible for setting up the internal terrain for a parasitic infection (e.g., does the patient have achlorhydria, decreased pancreatic enzyme output, etc.?).

In my clinical practice, when electing not to use an antibiotic, I like to use high dosages of pancreatic enzymes (10X USP pancreatic enzymes, 750 to 1,000 mg, 10 to 20 minutes before meals or on an empty stomach) along with goldenseal root (*Hydrastis canadensis*). Proper treatment with either an antibiotic or a natural alternative requires proper monitoring by repeating multiple stool samples two weeks after therapy.

Using Berberine-Containing Plants to Fight Parasitic Infections

Goldenseal contains berberis alkaloids. Several other plants contain similar compounds and can be used interchangeably with goldenseal. These plants include barberry (*Berberis vulgaris*), Oregon grape (*Berberis aquifolium*), and goldthread (*Coptis chinensis*). Given the growing scarcity of goldenseal (it is an endangered species), it is perhaps more appropriate to use one of these alternative sources of berberine alkaloids.

Berberine is the most important berberis alkaloid. It has been extensively studied in both experimental and clinical settings for its antibiotic activity against most intestinal parasites. Berberine exhibits a broad spectrum of antibiotic activity and has shown antibiotic activity against bacteria, protozoa, and fungi, including *Staph sp., Strep. sp., Chlamydia sp., Corynebacterium diphtheria, E. coli, Salmonella typhi, Vibrio cholerae, Diplococcus pneumonia, Pseudomonas sp., Shigella dysenteriae, Entamoeba histolytica, Trichomonas vaginalis, Neisseria gonorrhoeae* and *meningitidis, Treponema pallidum, Giardia lamblia, Leishmania donovani,* and *Candida albicans.*[31–40]

Berberine's antibiotic action against some of these pathogens (disease-producing organisms) is actually stronger than that of commonly used antibiotics. Berberine-containing plants should be considered in infectious processes involving the above-mentioned organisms. Also Berberine's action in inhibiting candida prevents the overgrowth of yeast that is a common side effect of antibiotic use.

Anti-Infective Activity of Berberine In addition to direct antibiotic activity, berberine has been shown to inhibit the binding of bacteria to epithelial cells—the type of cells that line the gastrointestinal, respiratory, and genitourinary tract. Recent studies of berberine's ability to inhibit the adherence of group A streptococci to host cells have shown that certain antimicrobial agents in berberine can block the adherence of microorganisms to host cells at doses much lower than those needed to kill cells or to inhibit cell growth.[41]

Berberine's ability to inhibit the adhesion of streptococci to host cells works by several modes of action. First of all, berberine causes streptococci to lose lipoteichoic acid (LTA). LTA is the major substance responsible for the adhesion of the bacteria to host tissues. Berberine also prevents the adhesion of fibronectin (a glue-like substance secreted by the epithelial cell) to the streptococci, as well as dissolving already bound fibronectin.

The results of this study are quite significant. It raises many questions and forces researchers as well as practitioners to look at the treatment of bacterial infections in a new light. Is it better to utilize a substance with bactericidal or bacteriostatic actions over a substance that prevents the adherence of bacteria to host cells? Is the true value of botanicals with "anti-infective" actions a multifactorial effect on all aspects of infections from immune stimulation to antimicrobial and anti-adherence actions?

Berberine may also enhance the immune system; it has been shown to increase the blood supply to the spleen as well as stimulate white blood cells.[42,43] Specifically, berberine enhances a type of white blood cell known as the macrophage. Macrophages are responsible for engulfing and destroying bacteria, viruses, tumor cells, and other particulate matter. The combined effect of improving blood supply to the spleen and increasing macrophage activity translates into improved filtration of the blood and is consistent with the historical use of berberine-containing plants as "blood purifiers."

Clinical Use of Berberine-Containing Plants in Parasitic Infections   Berberine has shown significant success in the treatment of acute diarrhea in several clinical studies. In humans it has been found effective against diarrheas caused by *E. coli* (traveler's diarrhea), *Shigella dysenteriae* (shigellosis), *Salmonella paratyphi* (food poisoning), *B. Klebsiella, Giardia lamblia* (giardiasis), and *Vibrio cholerae* (cholera).[44-54] Studies of hamsters and rats have shown that berberine also has significant activity against *Entamoeba histolytica,* the causative organism of amebiasis—a common cause of diarrhea in areas of poor sanitation.[37,38]

It appears that berberine is effective in treating the majority of common gastrointestinal infections. The clinical studies have produced results with berberine comparable to standard antibiotics in most cases. In fact, in several studies' results with berberine were better than those for standard antibiotics.

For example, in a study of 65 children below five years of age with acute diarrhea caused by *E. coli, Shigella, Salmonella, Klebsiella, or Faecalis aerogenes,* those given berberine tannate (25 mg every six hours) responded better compared to standard antibiotic therapy.[48]

In another study, 40 children (ages 1 to 10 years) infected with the parasite giardia received either berberine (5 mg per kg body weight each day), the drug metronidazole (10 mg per kg body weight each day), or a placebo of vitamin B syrup in three divided doses. After six days, 48% of patients treated with berberine were symptom-free and, on stool analysis, 68% were giardia-free. In the metronidazole (Flagyl) group, 33% of patients were without symptoms and, on stool analysis, all were giardia-free. In comparison, 15% of patients on placebo were asymptomatic and, on stool analysis, 25% were giardia-free.[49] These results indicate that berberine was more effective than metronidazole in relieving symptoms at half the dose, but was less effective than the drug in clearing the organism from the intestines.

And finally, in a study of 200 adult patients with acute diarrhea, the subjects were given standard antibiotic treatment with or without berberine hydrochloride (150 mg per day). Results of the study indicated that the patients receiving berberine recovered more quickly.[50] An additional 30 cases of acute diarrhea were treated with berberine alone. Berberine arrested diarrhea in all of these cases with no mortality or toxicity.

Despite these results, due to the serious consequences of ineffectively treated infectious diarrhea, the best approach may be to use berberine-containing plants along with standard antibiotic therapy.

Much of berberine's effectiveness is undoubtedly due to its direct antimicrobial activity, however, it also has an effect in blocking the action of toxins produced by certain bacteria.[55,56] This toxin-blocking effect is most evident in diarrhea caused by enterotoxins such as cholera (*Vibrio cholerae*) and traveler's diarrhea (*E. coli*).[52-54]

Cholera is a serious disorder that needs standard therapy, however, traveler's diarrhea is usually self-limiting. Good results with berberine in the treatment of traveler's diarrhea have been obtained. In one study, patients with traveler's diarrhea randomly received 400 mg of berberine sulfate in a single dose or served as controls.[54] In treated patients, the mean stool volumes were significantly less than those of controls during three consecutive 8-hour periods after treatment. At 24 hours after treatment, significantly more treated patients stopped having diarrhea as compared to controls (42% versus 20%).

For those planning to travel to an underdeveloped country or an area of poor water quality or sanitation, the prophylactic use of berberine-containing herbs during, and one week prior to and after, the visit may be useful.

Dosage Recommendations for Goldenseal   The dosage of goldenseal should be based on berberine content. As there is a wide range of quality in herbal preparations, standardized extracts are preferred. Three times a day dosages for adults are as follows:

Dried root or as infusion (tea): 2 to 4 grams

Tincture (1:5): 6 to 12 ml (1½ to 3 tsp)

Fluid extract (1:1): 2 to 4 ml (½ to 1 tsp)

Solid (powdered dry) extract (4:1 or 8% to 12% alkaloid content): 250 to 500 mg

My dosage recommendations for pure berberine would be 25 to 50 mg, three times daily or a daily dosage of up to 150 mg. This dosage is consistent with the dosage range in the positive clinical studies. For children a dosage based on body weight is appropriate. The daily dosage would be the equivalent to 5 to 10 mg of berberine per kg (2.2 pounds) of body weight or roughly 50 to 100 mg of goldenseal root extract per kg (i.e., a 50-pound child would take 1,000 to 2,000 mg per day).

Berberine and berberine-containing plants are generally nontoxic at the recommended dosages, however, berberine-containing plants are not recommended for use during pregnancy and higher dosages may interfere with B-vitamin metabolism.[57]

Final Comments

An old-time naturopathic physician once told me, "Good health begins in the colon." There appears to be great wisdom in that statement. It can definitely be stated that without proper elimination of waste products there are serious repercussions to our health. Maintaining and/or attaining good colon health is straightforward: eat a high-fiber diet, drink plenty of water, seed and maintain health-promoting microflora, and take appropriate actions when there are problems.

6

Food Allergies

The recognition of food allergy was first recorded by the famous Greek physician Hippocrates, who observed that milk could cause gastric upset and hives (urticaria). He wrote, "To many this has been the commencement of a serious disease when they have merely taken twice in a day the same food which they have been in the custom of taking once."[1]

A food allergy occurs when there is an adverse reaction to the ingestion of a food. The reaction may or may not be mediated by the immune system. The reaction may be caused by a food protein, starch, or other food component, or by a contaminant found in the food (colorings, preservatives, etc.). A classic food allergy occurs when an ingested food molecule acts as an *antigen,* which is defined as a substance that can be bound by an antibody, and is bound by antibodies known as IgE. IgE then binds to specialized white blood cells known as *mast cells* and *basophils.* This binding causes the release of substances such as histamine, which cause swelling and inflammation.

Other words often used to refer to a food allergy include food hypersensitivity, food anaphylaxis, food idiosyncrasy, food intolerance, pharmacologic (drug-like) reaction to food, metabolic reaction to food, and food sensitivity. From a clinical perspective, naturopaths, clinical ecologists, and preventive- and nutrition-oriented physicians recognize two basic types of food allergies—cyclic and fixed. Cyclic allergies account for 80% to 90% of food allergies. The sensitivity is slowly developed by repetitive eating of a food. If the allergic food is avoided for a period of time (typically over four months), it may be reintroduced and tolerated unless it is again eaten too frequently. Fixed allergies occur whenever a food is eaten, no matter what the time span is between ingestions. Long-term avoidance may reestablish tolerance, but it is no guarantee.

Signs and Symptoms of Food Allergies

Food allergies have been implicated as a causative factor in a wide range of conditions; no part of the human body is immune from being a target cell or organ. The actual symptoms produced during an allergic response depend on the location of the immune-system activation, the mediators of inflammation involved, and the sensitivity of the tissues to specific mediators. As shown in Table 6.1, food allergies have been linked to many common symptoms and health conditions.

The number of people suffering from food allergies has increased dramatically during the last 15 years. Some physicians claim that food allergies are the leading cause of most undiagnosed symptoms and that at least 60% of the U.S. population suffers from symptoms associated with food reactions.[2] Theories of why the incidence has increased include increased stresses on the immune system (such as greater chemical pollution in the air, water,

Table 6.1 Symptoms and Diseases Commonly Associated with Food Allergies

System	Symptoms and Diseases
Gastrointestinal	canker sores, celiac disease, chronic diarrhea, stomach ulcer, gas, gastritis, irritable colon, malabsorption, ulcerative colitis
Genitourinary	bed-wetting, chronic bladder infections, kidney disease
Immune	chronic infections, frequent ear infections
Mental/Emotional	anxiety, depression, hyperactivity, inability to concentrate, insomnia, irritability, mental confusion, personality change, seizures
Musculoskeletal	bursitis, joint pain, low back pain
Respiratory	asthma, chronic bronchitis, wheezing
Skin	acne, eczema, hives, itching, skin rash
Miscellaneous	arrythmia, edema, fainting, fatigue, headache, hypoglycemia, itchy nose or throat, migraines, sinusitis

and food), earlier weaning and earlier introduction of solid foods to infants, genetic manipulation of plants resulting in food components with greater allergenic tendencies, and increased ingestion of fewer foods. Probably all of these and more have contributed to the increased frequency and severity of symptoms.

Food allergies, as well as respiratory tract allergies, are also characterized by the following signs:

Dark circles under the eyes (allergic shiners)

Puffiness under the eyes

Horizontal creases in the lower lid

Chronic non-cyclic fluid retention

Chronic swollen glands

It is often not clearly apparent that a symptom is due to a food allergy. This appears to be due to the body adapting to chronic exposure to allergic foods. According to Theron Randolph, M.D., the symptom process may involve the following three stages:

Stage 1—Hypersensitivity (pre-adapted): Obvious allergic response following exposure to allergic food.

Stage 2—Adaptive: Less recognizable response after eating the allergic food and an increase in chronic symptoms. This can be considered an addictive phase, since ingestion of the allergic food(s) may actually temporarily relieve symptoms. This stage typically involves food cravings and withdrawal responses. This is also known as *masked allergies.*

Stage 3—Maladaptive: The body is in a constant state of biochemical dysfunction. The allergic person is totally unaware of sensitivities as a cause of their ill health.[3]

What Causes Food Allergies?

It is well-documented that food allergy is often inherited. When both parents have allergies, there is a 67% chance that the children will also have allergies. Where only one parent is allergic, the chance of a child being prone to allergies drops to 33%.[4] The actual expression of an allergy can be triggered by a variety of stressors that disrupt the immune system, such as physical and emotional trauma, excessive use of drugs, immunization reactions, excessive frequency of consumption of a specific food, and/or environmental toxins.

Most food allergies are mediated by the immune system as a result of interactions between ingested food, the digestive tract, white blood cells, and food-specific anti-bodies (immunoglobulins), such as IgE and IgG. Food molecules capable of being bound by antibodies are known as *antigens.* Food represents the largest antigenic challenge confronting the human immune system. When the immune system is activated by food antigens, white blood cells and antibodies cooperate in an immune response, which, under certain circumstances, can have negative effects.

There are five major families of antibodies: IgE, IgD, IgG, IgM, and IgA. IgE is involved primarily in the classic immediate reaction, while the others seem to be involved in delayed reactions, such as those seen in the cyclic type of food allergy. Although the function of the immune system is protection of the host from infections and cancer, abnormal immune responses can lead to tissue injury and disease (food allergy reactions being one expression). There are four distinct types of immune-mediated reactions: immediate hypersensitivity, cytotoxic reactions, immune-complex mediated reactions, and T-cell dependent reactions.

Immediate Hypersensitivity

With immediate hypersensitivity, the reactions occur in less than 2 hours after exposure to the allergen. Antigens bind to preformed IgE antibodies attached to the surface of the mast cell or the basophil and cause release of mediators: histamine, leukotrienes, and so on. A variety of allergic symptoms may result, depending on the location of the mast cell: In the nasal passages it causes sinus congestion; in the bronchioles, constriction (asthma); in the skin, hives and eczema; in the synovial cells that line the joints, arthritis; in the intestinal mucosa, inflammation with resulting malabsorption; and in the brain, headaches, loss of memory, and "spaciness." It has been estimated that immediate hypersensitivity reactions account for only 10% to 15% of food allergy reactions.[5]

Cytotoxic reactions

Cytotoxic reactions involve the binding of either IgG or IgM antibodies to cell-bound antigen. Antigen–antibody binding activates factors that result in the destruction of the cell to which the antigen is bound. Examples of tissue injury include immune hemolytic anemia. It has been estimated that at least 75% of all food allergy reactions are accompanied by cell destruction.[5]

Immune-Complex Mediated Reactions

Immune complexes are formed when antigens bind to antibodies. They are usually cleared from the circulation by the phagocytic system. However, if these complexes are deposited in tissues they can produce tissue injury. Two important factors that promote tissue injury are (1) increased quantities of circulating complexes and (2) the presence of histamine and other amines, which increase vascular permeability and favor the deposition of immune complexes in tissues.

These responses are of the delayed type, often occurring 2 hours after exposure. This type of allergy has been shown to involve IgG and IgG immune complexes. It is estimated that 80% of food allergy reactions involve IgG.[5]

T-Cell Dependent Reactions

This delayed type of reaction is mediated primarily by T-lymphocytes. It results when an allergen contacts the skin, respiratory tract, gastrointestinal tract, or some other body surface. Within 36 to 72 hours of contact, it can cause inflammation by stimulating sensitized T-cells. T-cell dependent reactions do not involve any antibodies. An example of this type of reaction is poison ivy (contact dermatitis).

Immune-System Disorders and Food Allergies

There are several immune-system disorders that can play a major role in food allergies. For example, some studies have shown that individuals with a tendency to develop asthma and eczema have abnormalities in the number and ratios of special white blood cells known as T-cells. Specifically, these individuals have nearly 50% more helper T-cells than nonallergic persons.[5] These cells help other white blood cells make antibodies.

An emerging theory suggests that individuals prone to asthma and eczema have a lower allergic set point. With more helper T-cells in circulation, the level of attack required to trigger an allergic response is lowered. Other T-cell abnormalities have been noted in patients with migraines and in asthmatic children; both groups commonly suffer from food allergies.[5]

Food-sensitive people usually have unusually low levels of secretory IgA.[6] IgA plays an important role on the lining of the mucosal membrane surfaces of the intestinal tract, where it helps protect against the entrance of foreign substances into the body. In other words, IgA acts as a barricade against the entry of food antigens. When there is a lack of IgA lining the intestines, the absorption of food allergens as well as microbial antigens increases dramatically. It has been suggested that even a short-term IgA deficiency predisposes to the development of allergy, especially during the first months of life.

There is also evidence that stress can impair immune function and lead to decreased secretory IgA.[7] These findings might explain the relationship that many observers report between food allergy and stress. During stress, food allergies tend to be more apparent.

Other Factors Triggering Food Allergies

Repetitious exposure to a food, improper digestion, and poor integrity of the intestinal barrier are additional factors that can lead to the development of food allergy. When properly chewed and digested, 98% of ingested proteins are absorbed as amino acids and small peptides. However, it has been well-documented that partially digested dietary protein can cross the intestinal barrier and be absorbed into the bloodstream. It then causes a food-allergic response, which can occur directly at the intestinal barrier, at distant sites, or throughout the body.

Gastric acidity and pancreatic enzymes limit the passage of organisms into the intestinal tract and are important in the digestion of protein. Low hydrochloric-acid and pancreatic-enzyme levels are associated with an increased incidence of intestinal infections and increased circulating antibodies to foods. It is often necessary to support the individual with food allergies with supplemental levels of hydrochloric acid and/or pancreatic enzymes because incompletely digested proteins can impair the immune system, leading to long-term allergies.

In addition to lack of digestive factors, other causes of an increased intestinal absorption of large protein molecules include immaturity of the gastrointestinal system, abnormal bacteria in the gut, vitamin A deficiency, inflammation of the intestinal tract, intestinal ulceration, and diarrhea. Proper functioning of the liver is also very important due to its role in removing foreign proteins.

Table 6.2 Mechanisms Responsible for
Pseudo-allergic Reactions

- Increased production of inflammatory mediators
- Activation of platelets, resulting in serotonin release
- Enhanced reactivity of mast cells and/or basophils to various triggering stimuli
- Excessive intake of histamine-containing foods: sausage, sauerkraut, tuna, wine, preserves, spinach, tomato
- Excessive intake of histamine-releasing foods: mollusks, crustaceans, strawberry, tomato, chocolate, protease-containing fruits (bananas, papaya), lectin-containing nuts, peptones, alcohol
- Intolerance to foods containing vasoactive amines: tyramine (cabbage, cheese, citrus, seafood, potato), serotonin (banana), phenylethylamine (chocolate)

Nonimmunological Mechanisms

Many adverse reactions to foods are not triggered by the immune system. Instead, the reaction is caused by inflammatory mediators (prostaglandins, leukotrienes, SRS-A, serotonin, platelet-activating factor, histamine, kinins, etc.). Foods may also produce a pseudo-allergic reaction due to histamine content or histamine-releasing effects and reactions to compounds in foods known as *biogenic amines,* including such compounds as tyramine, serotonin, and polyamines.(See Table 6.2.)

Diagnosis of Food Allergies

Two basic categories of tests are commonly used: (1) food challenge and (2) laboratory methods. Each has its advantages. Food-challenge methods require no additional expense, but do require a great deal of motivation. Laboratory procedures, such as blood tests, can provide immediate identification of suspected allergens, but are more expensive.

Food Challenge

Many physicians believe that oral food challenge is the best way of diagnosing food sensitivities. There are two broad categories of food challenge testing: (1) elimination (also known as oligoantigenic) diet, followed by food reintroduction, and (2) pure water fast, followed by food challenge. A note of caution, food-challenge testing should *not* be used in people with symptoms that are potentially life-threatening (such as airway constriction or severe allergic reactions).

In the elimination-diet method, the person is placed on a limited diet; commonly eaten foods are eliminated and replaced with either hypoallergenic foods and foods rarely eaten or special hypoallergenic formulas.[8,9] The fewer the allergic foods, the greater the ease of establishing a diagnosis with an elimination diet. The standard elimination diet consists of lamb, chicken, potato, rice, banana, apple, and a cabbage-family vegetable (cabbage, brussels sprouts, broccoli, etc.). There are variations of the elimination diet that are suitable, however, it is extremely important that no allergenic foods be consumed.

The individual stays on this limited diet for at least one week and up to one month. If the symptoms are related to food sensitivity, they will typically disappear by the fifth or sixth day of the diet. If the symptoms do not disappear, it is possible that a reaction to a food in the elimination diet is responsible, in which case an even more restricted diet must be utilized.

After one week, individual foods are reintroduced. Methods range from reintroducing only a single food every two days, to one every one or two meals. Usually after the one week "cleansing" period, the patient will develop an increased sensitivity to offending foods.

Reintroduction of sensitive foods will typically produce a more severe or recognizable symptom than before. A careful, detailed, record must be maintained that describes when foods were reintroduced and what symptoms appeared upon reintroduction.[10] It can be very useful to track the wrist pulse during reintroduction, as pulse changes may occur when an allergic food is consumed.[11]

For many people, elimination diets offer the most viable means of detection. Because one can sometimes dramatically experience the effects of food reactions, motivation to eliminate the food can be high. The downside of this procedure is that it is time-consuming and requires discipline and motivation.

A refinement which often yields better results than the simple elimination diet is the five-day water fast with subsequent food challenge. Proponents of this approach believe that it is necessary for the patient to fast for at least five days in order to clear the body of allergic responses.[12] During the fast, "withdrawal" symptoms will likely be experienced. These symptoms will usually subside by the fourth day. As in the elimination diet, symptoms caused by food allergy will diminish or be eliminated after the fourth day.

After the five-day fast, individual foods are reintroduced one at a time, with the monitoring of symptoms and pulse. Due to the hyper-reactive state, symptoms tend to be more acute and pronounced than before the fast. This method can produce dramatic results, greatly motivating avoidance of the offending foods.

This method is advisable only for people who are physically and mentally capable of a five-day water fast. Close monitoring by a physician with experience in fasting is highly recommended. At times, careful interpretation of results is needed, due to the occurrence of delayed reactions.

Laboratory Methods

Laboratory methods for detecting food allergies consist of either skin or blood tests.

Skin Tests   It must be pointed out that the skin-prick test or skin-scratch test commonly employed by many allergists only tests for IgE-mediated allergies. Because only about 10% to 15% of all food allergies are mediated by IgE, this test is of little value in diagnosing most food allergies. Nonetheless, skin tests are often performed.

Food extracts are placed on the patient's skin with a scratch or prick. If the patient is allergic to the food, a welt will form immediately as the allergen reacts with IgE-sensitized cells in the patient's skin.

Blood Tests   Despite a tremendous amount of scientific support, the diagnosis of food allergy by blood testing is still somewhat controversial in conventional medical settings. These tests are convenient, but can range in cost from a modest $130 to an extravagant $1,200. A variety of blood tests are available to physicians with the RAST (radio-allergo-sorbent test) and the ELISA (enzyme-linked immunosorbent assay) test appearing to be the best laboratory methods currently available. In my clinical practice, I tend to favor the ELISA tests, which determine both IgE- and IgG-mediated food allergies. Laboratories that I would recommend for this analysis are National BioTech Laboratory (1-800-846-6285) and Meridian Valley Clinical Laboratory (1-206-859-8700). These laboratories offer IgE and IgG food-allergy panel tests for over 100 different foods; the tests come with detailed dietary instructions and are reasonably priced at about $130.

Dealing with Food Allergies

Avoiding Allergenic Foods

The simplest and most effective method of treating food allergies is through avoidance of allergenic foods. Elimination of the offending antigens from the diet will begin to alleviate associated symptoms after the body has cleared itself of the antigen–antibody complexes and after the intestinal tract has transited out any remaining food (usually three to five days). Avoidance means not only avoiding the food in its most identifiable state (e.g., eggs in an omelet), but also in its hidden state (e.g., eggs in bread). For severe reactions, closely related foods with similar antigenic components may also need to be eliminated (e.g., rice and millet in patients with severe wheat allergy).

However, avoiding allergenic foods may not be practical, for several reasons:

1. Common allergenic foods such as wheat, corn, and soy are found as components of many processed foods.

2. When eating away from home, it is often difficult to determine what ingredients are used in purchased foods and prepared meals.

3. There has been a dramatic increase in the number of foods that single individuals are allergic to. This condition represents a syndrome that is possibly indicative of broad immune-system dysfunction. It may be difficult (psychologically, socially, and nutritionally) to eliminate a large number of common foods from a person's diet.

A possible solution is the Rotary Diversified Diet.

Rotary Diversified Diet

Many experts believe that the key to the dietary control of food allergies is the *Rotary Diversified Diet*. The diet was first developed by Dr. Herbert J. Rinkel in 1934.[13] The diet is made up of a highly varied selection of foods, which are eaten in a definite rotation, or order, to prevent the formation of new allergies and to control preexisting ones. Tolerated foods are eaten at regularly spaced intervals of four to seven days. For example, if a person has wheat on Monday, she will have to wait until Friday to have anything with wheat in it again. This approach is based on the principle that infrequent consumption of tolerated foods is not likely to induce new allergies or increase any mild allergies, even in highly sensitized and immune-compromised individuals. As tolerance for eliminated foods returns, they may be added back into the rotation schedule without reactivation of the allergy (this, of course, applies only to cyclic food allergies—fixed allergenic foods may never be eaten again).

It is not simply a matter of rotating tolerated foods; food families must also be rotated. Foods, whether animal or vegetable, come in families. The reason it is important to rotate food families is that foods in one family can cross-react with allergenic foods. Steady consumption of foods that are members of the same family can lead to allergies. Food families need not be as strictly rotated as individual foods. It is usually recommended to avoid eating members of the same food family two days in a row. Table 6.3 lists family classifications for edible plants and animals while a simplified four-day rotation diet plan is provided in Table 6.4.

Table 6.3   Edible Plant and Animal Kingdom Taxonomic List

Vegetables

Legumes	Mustard	Parsley	Potato	Grass
Beans	Broccoli	Anise	Chili	Barley
Cocoa bean	Brussels sprout	Caraway	Eggplant	Corn
Lentil	Cabbage	Carrot	Peppers	Oat
Licorice	Cauliflower	Celery	Potatoes	Rice
Peanut	Mustard	Coriander	Tomato	Rye
Peas	Radish	Cumin	Tobacco	Wheat
Soybean	Turnip	Parsley		
Tamarind	Watercress			

Lily	Laurel	Sunflower	Beet	Buckwheat
Asparagus	Avocado	Artichoke	Beet	Buckwheat
Chives	Camphor	Lettuce	Chard	Rhubarb
Garlic	Cinnamon	Sunflower	Spinach	
Leek				
Onions				

Fruits

Gourds	Plums	Citrus	Cashew	Nuts
Cantaloupe	Almond	Grapefruit	Cashew	Brazil nut
Cucumber	Apricot	Lemon	Mango	Pecan
Honeydew	Cherry	Lime	Pistachio	Walnut
Melons	Peach	Mandarin		
Pumpkin	Plum	Orange		
Squash	Persimmon	Tangerine		
Zucchini				

Beech	Banana	Palm	Grape	Pineapple
Beechnut	Arrowroot	Coconut	Grape	Pineapple
Chestnut	Banana	Date	Raisin	
Chinquapin nut	Plantain	Date sugar		

Rose	Birch	Apple	Blueberry	Pawpaw
Blackberry	Filberts	Apple	Blueberry	Papaya
Loganberry	Hazelnuts	Pear	Cranberry	Pawpaw
Raspberry		Quince	Huckleberry	
Rosehips				
Strawberry				

Continued

Table 6.3 Edible Plant and Animal Kingdom Taxonomic List
(continued)

| | | Animals | | |
Mammals (Meat/Milk)	Birds (Meat/Eggs)	Fish	Crustaceans	Mollusks
Cow	Chicken	Catfish	Crab	Abalone
Goat	Duck	Cod	Crayfish	Clams
Pig	Goose	Flounder	Lobster	Mussels
Rabbit	Hen	Halibut	Prawn	Oysters
Sheep	Turkey	Mackerel	Shrimp	Scallops
		Salmon		
		Sardine		
		Snapper		
		Trout		
		Tuna		

Table 6.4 Four-day Rotation Diet

Food Family	Food
Day 1	
Citrus	Lemon, orange, grapefruit, lime, tangerine, kumquat, citron
Banana	Banana, plantain, arrowroot (musa)
Palm	Coconut, date, date sugar
Parsley	Carrots, parsnips, celery, celery seed, celeriac, anise, dill, fennel, cumin, parsley, coriander, caraway
Spices	Black and white pepper, peppercorn, nutmeg, mace
Subucaya	Brazil nut
Bird	All fowl and game birds, including chicken, turkey, duck, goose, guinea, pigeon, quail, pheasant, eggs
Juices	Juices (preferably fresh) may be made and used from any fruits and vegetables listed above, in any combination desired, without adding sweeteners.
Day 2	
Grape	All varieties of grapes, raisins
Pineapple	Juice-pack, water-pack, or fresh

Table 6.4 Four-day Rotation Diet *(continued)*

Food Family	Food
Rose	Strawberry, raspberry, blackberry, loganberry, rosehips
Gourd	Watermelon, cucumber, cantaloupe, pumpkin, squash, other melons, zucchini, pumpkin or squash seeds
Beet	Beet, spinach, chard
Legume	Pea, black-eyed pea, dry beans, green beans, carob, soybeans, lentils, licorice, peanut, alfalfa
Cashew	Cashew, pistachio, mango
Birch	Filberts, hazelnuts
Flaxseed	Flaxseed
Swine	All pork products
Mollusks	Abalone, snail, squid, clam, mussel, oyster, scallop
Crustaceans	Crab, crayfish, lobster, prawn, shrimp
Juices	Juices (preferably fresh) may be made from any fruits, berries, or vegetables listed above and used without added sweeteners, in any combination desired, including fresh alfalfa and some legumes
Day 3	
Apple	Apple, pear, quince
Gooseberry	Currant, gooseberry
Buckwheat	Buckwheat, rhubarb
Aster	Lettuce, chicory, endive, escarole, globe artichoke, dandelion, sunflower seeds, tarragon
Potato	Potato, tomato, eggplant, peppers (red and green), chili pepper, paprika, cayenne, ground cherries
Lily (onion)	Onion, garlic, asparagus, chives, beets
Spurge	Tapioca
Herb	Basil, savory, sage, oregano, horehound, catnip, spearmint, peppermint, thyme, marjoram, lemon balm
Walnut	English walnut, black walnut, pecan, hickory nut, butternut
Pedalium	Sesame
Beech	Chestnut
Saltwater fish	Herring, anchovy, cod, sea bass, sea trout, mackerel, tuna, swordfish, flounder, sole
Freshwater fish	Sturgeon, salmon, whitefish, bass, perch

Continued

Table 6.4   Four-day Rotation Diet *(continued)*

Food Family	Food
Juices	Juices (preferably fresh) may be made from any fruits and vegetables listed above and used without added sweeteners, in any combination
Day 4	
Plum	Plum, cherry, peach, apricot, nectarine, almond, wild cherry
Blueberry	Blueberry, huckleberry, cranberry, wintergreen
Pawpaws	Pawpaw, papaya, papain
Mustard	Mustard, turnip, radish, horseradish, watercress, cabbage, Chinese cabbage, broccoli, cauliflower, Brussels sprouts, kale, kohlrabi, rutabaga
Laurel	Avocado, cinnamon, bay leaf, sassafras, cassia buds or bark
Sweet potato or yam	
Grass	Wheat, corn, rice, oats, barley, rye, wild rice, cane, millet, sorghum, bamboo sprouts
Orchid	Vanilla
Protea	Macadamia nut
Conifer	Pine nut
Fungus	Mushrooms and yeast (brewer's yeast, etc.)
Bovid	Milk products—butter, cheese, yogurt, beef and milk products, oleomargarine, lamb
Juices	Juices (preferably fresh) may be made from any fruits and vegetables listed above and used without added sweeteners, in any combination desired.

Final Comments

While there is no known simple "cure" for food allergies, a number of measures will help to avoid and lessen symptoms and can correct the underlying causes. First, all allergenic foods should be identified using one of the methods discussed above. After identifying allergenic foods, the best approach is clearly avoidance of all major allergens, and rotation of all other foods for at least the first few months. As one improves, the dietary restrictions can be relaxed, although some individuals may always require a rotation diet indefinitely. For strongly allergenic foods, all members of the food family should be avoided.

7

Dietary Guidelines

A primary dietary guideline was covered in the preceding chapter—identify and control your food allergies. Beyond that my recommendations for a diet for someone with digestive disturbances mirrors my recommendations for most patients. There are two additional recommendations, however, that I often stress to patients with digestive disturbances: (1) get a juice extractor and drink 16 to 24 ounces of fresh juice per day and (2) consider food combining.

Why Juice?

Fresh juice, the liquid extracted from fresh fruits and vegetables, provides high quality nutrition that is easily absorbed. Fresh juice is referred to as a "live" food because it contains active enzymes. Enzymes are extremely sensitive to heat; they are destroyed during cooking and pasteurization.

The body process that utilizes the greatest level of energy is digestion. One of the key energy-enhancing benefits of fresh juice is that it is in a highly digestible form. When you eat, the digestive system works very hard at separating out the juice from the fiber. When you drink fresh juice, the juice extractor has already performed this function. Fresh juice and other "live" foods contain digestive enzymes that break down foods in the digestive tract, thereby sparing the body's valuable digestive enzymes. This action is referred to as the "Law of Adaptive Secretion of Digestive Enzymes."[1]

According to this law, if some of the food is digested by the enzymes contained in the food, the body will secrete less of its own enzymes. This allows vital energy in the body to be shifted from digestion to other bodily functions, such as repair and rejuvenation. Fresh juices require very little energy to digest. In as little as 5 minutes they begin to be absorbed. In contrast, a big meal of steak and potatoes may sit in the stomach for hours. If a meal is composed entirely from cooked (no enzyme) foods, most of the body's energy is directed at digestion.

Fresh juice provides easily-digested protein, carbohydrates, essential fatty acids, and vitamins and minerals. Fresh juice also provides a wide assortment of compounds that are extremely beneficial to health, including enzymes; pigments such as carotenes, chlorophyll, and flavonoids; and numerous accessory components that help to protect our cells from damage.

What to Juice

Although some specific juices have been shown to offer benefits in certain health conditions (e.g., cabbage juice in the treatment of peptic ulcers), in general, you should juice a wide assortment of fruits and vegetables rather than relying too heavily on any one juice. This ensures that a broad range of beneficial substances are being delivered to the body as well as protecting against developing food allergies to a too frequently consumed food.

Supplementing your juices with medicinal herbs and spices can provide great benefit. One of my favorite additions to juice is fresh ginger—a plant that demonstrates many positive effects on the gastrointestinal tract. One interesting aspect of ginger is its ability to simultaneously improve gastric motility while exerting antispasmodic effects. This is consistent with its use as a gastrointestinal tonic.

A clue to ginger's success in eliminating gastrointestinal distress is offered by some recent double-blind studies which demonstrated that ginger is very effective in preventing the symptoms of motion sickness, especially seasickness.[2-4] In fact, in one study ginger was shown to be far superior to Dramamine, a commonly used drug for motion sickness.[2] Ginger reduces all symptoms associated with motion sickness, including dizziness, nausea, vomiting, and cold sweats.

Historically, ginger also has been used for the treatment of nausea and vomiting of pregnancy. Recently, the benefit of ginger was confirmed in the most severe form of nausea and vomiting of pregnancy (hyperemesis gravidarum),[5] a condition that usually requires hospitalization. Ginger root powder at a dose of 250 mg, four times a day brought about a significant reduction in both the severity of the nausea and the number of attacks of vomiting.

Other examples of delicious and healthful additions to juice include garlic, parsley, basil, capsicum (red pepper), onions, and dandelion greens or roots.

Food Combining

Food combining is based on the theory that our bodies find it difficult to digest and assimilate numerous types of food consumed at one meal. I have read many of the explanations trying to justify this concept and most of them do not stand up to scientific reasoning. However, the bottom line is that some people, especially people suffering from digestive disturbances, do seem to function better when they adhere to the rather simple guidelines of food combining that I have summarized below:

1. Never eat an animal protein source with starches (breads, grains, potatoes, etc.).
2. Never eat more than one animal protein source per meal (e.g., no ham with eggs).
3. Combine protein with vegetables.
4. Combine starches with vegetables.
5. Always eat fruits alone or in combination with other fruits.
6. Do not eat refined sugar with any other food (if at all).
7. Do not overeat; consume moderate portions or more frequent small portions.

Constructing a Healthful Diet

The American Dietetic Association (ADA) in conjunction with the American Diabetes Association and other groups, has developed the *Exchange System,* a convenient tool for the rapid estimation of the calorie, protein, fat, and carbohydrate content of a diet. Originally used in designing dietary recommendations for diabetics, the exchange method is now used in the calculation and design of virtually all therapeutic diets. Unfortunately, the ADA exchange plan does not place a strong enough focus on the *quality* of food choices.

The Healthy Exchange System presented here (as well as in *The Healing Power of Foods*) is a superior version because it emphasizes more healthful food choices and focuses on unprocessed, whole foods. The diet is prescribed by allotting the number of exchanges allowed per list for one day. There are seven exchange lists, however, the milk and meat lists should be considered optional:

The Healthy Exchange System
 Vegetables
 Fruits
 Breads, Cereals, and Starchy Vegetables
 Legumes
 Fats and Oils
 Milk
 Meats, Fish, Cheese, and Eggs

Because all food portions within each exchange list provide approximately the same amount of calories, proteins, fats, and carbohydrates per serving it is easy to construct a diet consisting of the recommended percentages of:

Carbohydrates:	65% to 75% of total calories
Fats:	15% to 25% of total calories
Protein:	10% to 15% of total calories
Dietary fiber:	at least 50 grams

Of the carbohydrates ingested, 90% should be complex carbohydrates or naturally occurring sugars. Intake of refined carbohydrates and concentrated sugars (including honey, pasteurized fruit juices, and dried fruit, as well as sugar and white flour) should be limited to less than 10% of the total calorie intake.

Constructing a diet that meets these recommendations is simple using the exchange lists. In addition, the recommendations ensure a high intake of vital whole foods, particularly vegetables, which are rich in nutritional value.

How Many Calories Do You Need?

In determining caloric needs, it is necessary to first determine your ideal body weight. The most popular height and weight charts are the tables of "desirable weight" provided by the Metropolitan Life Insurance Company. The most recent edition of these tables, published in 1983, gives weight ranges for men and women at one inch increments of height for three body frame sizes (see Table 7.1).

Determining Frame Size and Activity Level

To make a simple determination of your frame size, extend your arm and bend your forearm upward at a 90-degree angle. Keep your fingers straight and turn the inside of your wrist away from your body. Place the thumb and index finger of your other hand on the two prominent bones on either side of your elbow. Measure the space between your fingers with a tape measure. Compare the measurement with the measurements for medium-framed individuals shown in Table 7.2. A lower reading indicates a small frame; a higher reading indicates a large frame.

After determining your desirable weight in pounds, convert it to kilograms by dividing it by 2.2. Next, take this

Table 7.1 1983 Metropolitan Life Insurance
Height and Weight Table

Height	Small Frame	Medium Frame	Large Frame
Men			
5'2"	128–134	131–141	138–150
5'3"	130–136	133–143	140–153
5'4"	132–138	135–145	142–156
5'5"	134–140	137–148	144–160
5'6"	136–142	139–151	146–164
5'7"	138–145	142–154	149–168
5'8"	140–148	145–157	152–172
5'9"	142–151	148–160	155–176
5'10"	144–154	151–163	158–180
5'11"	146–157	154–166	161–184
6'0"	149–160	157–170	164–188
6'1"	152–164	160–174	168–192
6'2"	155–168	164–178	172–197
6'3"	158–172	167–182	176–202
6'4"	162–176	171–187	181–207
Women			
4'10"	102–111	109–121	118–131
4'11"	103–113	111–123	120–134
5'0"	104–115	113–126	122–137
5'1"	106–118	115–129	125–140
5'2"	108–121	118–132	128–143
5'3"	111–124	121–135	131–147
5'4"	114–127	124–138	134–151
5'5"	117–130	127–141	137–155
5'6"	120–133	130–144	140–159
5'7"	123–136	133–147	143–163
5'8"	126–139	136–150	146–167
5'9"	129–142	139–153	149–170
5'10"	132–145	142–156	152–173
5'11"	135–148	145–159	155–176
6'0"	138–151	148–162	158–179

*Weights for adults ages 25 to 59 years based on lowest mortality.
Weight in pounds according to frame size in indoor clothing (5 pounds for men and 3 pounds for women) wearing shoes with 1-inch heels

Table 7.2 Measurements for Medium-Framed Individuals

	Height in 1-inch heels	Elbow breadth
Men		
	5'2" to 5'3"	2½" to 2⅞"
	5'4" to 5'7"	2⅝" to 2⅞"
	5'8" to 5'11"	2¾" to 3"
	6'0" to 6'3"	2¾" to 3⅛"
	6'4"	2⅞" to 3¼"
Women		
	4'10" to 5'3"	2¼" to 2½"
	5'4" to 5'11"	2⅜" to 2⅝"
	6'0"	2½" to 2¾"

number and multiply it by the following calories, depending upon your activity level:

Little physical activity:	30 calories
Light physical activity:	35 calories
Moderate physical activity:	40 calories
Heavy physical activity:	45 calories

Weight (in Kg) × Activity Level = Approximate Calorie Requirements

_____ × _____ = _____

Examples of Exchange Recommendations

1,500 Calorie Vegan Diet

Vegetables: 5 servings

Fruits: 2 servings

Breads, Cereals, and Starchy Vegetables: 9 servings

Beans: 2.5 servings

Fats: 4 servings

The above diet would result in an intake of approximately 1,500 calories per day, of which 67% are derived from complex carbohydrates and naturally occurring sugars, 18% from fat, and 15% from protein. The protein intake is entirely from plant sources, but still provides approximately 55 grams; this number is well above the recommended daily allowance of protein intake for someone requiring 1,500 calories. At least half of the fat servings should be from nuts, seeds, and other whole foods from the fat and oils exchange list. The dietary fiber intake would be approximately 31 to 74.5 grams.

1,500 Calorie Omnivore Diet

Vegetables: 5 servings

Fruits: 2.5 servings

Breads, Cereals, and Starchy Vegetables: 6 servings

Beans: 1 serving

Fats: 5 servings

Milk: 1 serving

Meats, Fish, Cheese, and Eggs: 2 servings

Percentage of calories as carbohydrates: 67%

Percentage of calories as fats: 18%

Percentage of calories as protein: 15%

Protein content: 61 g (75% from plant sources)

Dietary fiber content: 19.5 to 53.5 g

2,000 Calorie Vegan Diet

Vegetables: 5.5 servings

Fruits: 2 servings

Breads, Cereals, and Starchy Vegetables: 11 servings
Beans: 5 servings
Fats: 8 servings
Percentage of calories as carbohydrates: 67%
Percentage of calories as fats: 18%
Percentage of calories as protein: 15%
Protein content: 79 g
Dietary fiber content: 48.5 to 101.5 g

2,000 Calorie Omnivore Diet
Vegetables: 5 servings
Fruits: 2.5 servings
Breads, Cereals, and Starchy Vegetables: 13 servings
Beans: 2 servings
Fats: 7 servings
Milk: 1 serving
Meats, Fish, Cheese, and Eggs: 2 servings
Percentage of calories as carbohydrates: 66%
Percentage of calories as fats: 19%
Percentage of calories as protein: 15%
Protein content: 78 g (72% from plant sources)
Dietary fiber content: 32.5 to 88.5 g

2,500 Calorie Vegan Diet
Vegetables: 8 servings
Fruits: 3 servings
Breads, Cereals, and Starchy Vegetables: 17 servings
Beans: 5 servings
Fats: 8 servings
Percentage of calories as carbohydrates: 69%

Percentage of calories as fats: 15%
Percentage of calories as protein: 16%
Protein content: 101 g
Dietary fiber content: 33 to 121 g

2,500 Calorie Omnivore Diet
Vegetables: 8 servings
Fruits: 3.5 servings
Breads, Cereals, and Starchy Vegetables: 17 servings
Beans: 2 servings
Fats: 8 servings
Milk: 1 serving
Meats, Fish, Cheese, and Eggs: 3 servings
    Percentage of calories as carbohydrates: 66%
    Percentage of calories as fats: 18%
    Percentage of calories as protein: 16%
    Protein content: 102 g (80% from plant sources)
    Dietary fiber content: 40.5 to 116.5 g

3,000 Calorie Vegan Diet
Vegetables: 10 servings
Fruits: 4 servings
Breads, Cereals, and Starchy Vegetables: 17 servings
Beans: 6 servings
Fats: 10 servings
    Percentage of calories as carbohydrates: 70%
    Percentage of calories as fats: 16%
    Percentage of calories as protein: 14%
    Protein content: 116 g
    Dietary fiber content: 50 to 84 g

3,000 Calorie Omnivore Diet

 Vegetables: 10 servings

 Fruits: 3 servings

 Breads, Cereals, and Starchy Vegetables: 20 servings

 Beans: 2 servings

 Fats: 10 servings

 Milk: 1 serving

 Meats, Fish, Cheese, and Eggs: 3 servings

  Percentage of calories as carbohydrates: 67%

  Percentage of calories as fats: 18%

  Percentage of calories as protein: 15%

  Protein content: 116 g (81% from plant sources)

  Dietary fiber content: 45 to 133 g

Note: Use these recommendations as the basis for calculating other calorie diets. For example, for a 4,000 calorie diet add the 2,500 to the 1,500. For a 1,000 calorie diet divide the 2,000 calorie diet in half.

The Healthy Exchange Lists

Vegetables

Vegetables provide the broadest range of nutrients of any food class. They are rich sources of vitamins, minerals, carbohydrates, and protein. For example, the percentage of protein (dry weight) ranges from 11% for potatoes to over 40% for cabbage family vegetables, spinach, and turnip greens. The little fat that vegetables contain is in the form of essential fatty acids. Vegetables provide high quantities of other valuable health-promoting substances, especially fiber and carotenes. In Latin, the word *vegetable* means "to enliven or animate." Vegetables give us life. Accumulated evidence shows that vegetables can prevent as well as treat many diseases.

Vegetables should play a major role in the diet. The U.S. National Academy of Science, the U.S. Department of Health and Human Services, and the National Cancer Institute recommend that Americans consume a minimum of three to five servings of vegetables per day. Unfortunately, less than 11% of all Americans achieve this goal.

Vegetables are the richest sources of antioxidant compounds that provide protection against free radicals. Free radicals are highly reactive molecules that can bind to and destroy cellular components. Free radicals have also been shown to be responsible for the initiation of many diseases including the two biggest killers of Americans—heart disease and cancer. Diabetics appear to be especially sensitive to the negative effects of free radicals. Increasing the intake of dietary antioxidants—such as carotenes, chlorophyll, vitamin C, sulfur-containing compounds, vitamin E, and selenium—by increasing the amounts of vegetables in the diet is essential in the long-term treatment of diabetes.

The best way to consume many vegetables is in their fresh, raw form. In their fresh form, many of the nutrients and health-promoting compounds of vegetables are provided in much higher concentrations. Drinking fresh vegetable juices is a phenomenal way to make sure you are achieving your daily quota of vegetables.

When cooking vegetables it is very important that they not be overcooked. Overcooking will not only result in loss of important nutrients, it will also alter the flavor of the vegetable. Light steaming, baking, and quick stir-frying are the best ways to cook vegetables. Do not boil vegetables unless you are making soup, because many of the nutrients will be left in the water. If fresh vegetables are not available, frozen vegetables are preferred over their canned counterparts.

Vegetables are fantastic "diet" foods because they are very high in nutritional value and low in calories. In the list below you will notice there is also a list of "free" vegetables. These vegetables are termed "free foods" and can be eaten in any desired amount because the calories they contain are offset by the number of calories your body burns in the process of digestion. If you are trying to lose weight, these foods are especially valuable as they help to keep you feeling satisfied between meals.

The list below shows the vegetables to use for one vegetable exchange. One cup of cooked vegetables or fresh vegetable juice or 2 cups of raw vegetables equals one exchange. Please notice that starchy vegetables such as potatoes and yams are included under Breads, Cereals, and Starchy Vegetables.

Vegetables

>   Artichoke (1 medium)
>
>   Asparagus
>
>   Bean sprouts
>
>   Beets
>
>   Broccoli
>
>   Brussels sprouts
>
>   Carrots
>
>   Cauliflower
>
>   Eggplant
>
>   Greens:
>
> >   Beet
> >
> >   Chard
> >
> >   Collard
> >
> >   Dandelion
> >
> >   Kale

Mustard
Spinach
Turnip
Mushrooms
Okra
Onions
Rhubarb
Rutabaga
Sauerkraut
String beans, green or yellow
Summer squash
Tomatoes, tomato juice, vegetable juice cocktail
Zucchini

Free Vegetables (may be consumed as often as desired, especially raw)
Alfalfa sprouts
Bell peppers
Bok choy
Cabbage
Chicory
Celery
Chinese cabbage
Cucumber
Endive
Escarole
Lettuce
Parsley
Radishes
Spinach
Turnips
Watercress

Fruits

Fruits are a rich source of many beneficial compounds and regular fruit consumption has been shown to offer significant protection against many chronic degenerative diseases including cancer, heart disease, cataracts, and strokes. Fruits make excellent snacks because they contain fructose or fruit sugar, which is absorbed slowly into the bloodstream thereby allowing the body time to utilize it. Fruits are also excellent sources of vitamins and minerals as well as health-promoting fiber compounds. However, fruits are not as nutrient dense as vegetables because they are typically higher in calories. That is why vegetables are favored over fruits in weight-loss plans and overall healthful diets.

If you are a diabetic, be careful to monitor your blood glucose levels after drinking any fruit juice because it may necessitate changing the dosage of your medication.

Fruits
Each of the following equals one exchange:

> Fresh juice, 1 cup (8 oz)
>
> Pasteurized juice, ⅔ cup
>
> Apple, 1 large
>
> Applesauce (unsweetened), 1 cup
>
> Apricots, fresh, 4 medium
>
> Apricots, dried, 8 halves
>
> Banana, 1 medium
>
> Berries:
>
>> Blackberries, 1 cup
>>
>> Blueberries, 1 cup
>>
>> Cranberries, 1 cup
>>
>> Raspberries, 1 cup
>>
>> Strawberries, 1½ cups

Cherries, 20 large

Dates, 4

Figs, fresh, 2

Figs, dried, 2

Grapefruit, 1

Grapes, 20

Mango, 1 small

Melons:

    Cantaloupe, ½ small

    Honeydew, ¼ medium

    Watermelon, 2 cups

Nectarines, 2 small

Orange, 1 large

Papaya, 1½ cups

Peaches, 2 medium

Persimmons, native, 2 medium

Pineapple, 1 cup

Plums, 4 medium

Prunes, 4 medium

Prune juice, ½ cup

Raisins, 4 tbsp

Tangerines, 2 medium

Additional fruit exchanges (no more than one per day):

    Honey, 1 tbsp

    Jams, jellies, preserves, 1 tbsp

    Sugar, 1 tbsp

Breads, Cereals, and Starchy Vegetables

Breads, cereals, and starchy vegetables are classified as complex carbohydrates. Chemically complex carbohydrates are made up of long chains of simple carbohydrates or sugars. This means that the body has to break down the large sugar chains into simple sugars. The sugar from complex carbohydrates enters the bloodstream slowly, which means that blood sugar levels and appetite are better controlled.

Complex carbohydrate foods such as breads, cereals, and starchy vegetables are higher in fiber and nutrients but lower in calories than foods high in simple sugars such as cakes and candies. Choose whole grain products (e.g., whole grain breads, whole grain flour products, brown rice, etc.) over their processed counterparts (white bread, white flour products, white rice, etc.). Whole grains provide substantially more nutrients and health-promoting properties. Whole grains are a major source of complex carbohydrates, dietary fiber, minerals, and B vitamins. The protein content and quality of whole grains is greater than that of refined grains. Diets rich in whole grains have been shown to be protective against the development of chronic degenerative diseases, especially cancer, heart disease, diabetes, varicose veins, and diseases of the colon including colon cancer, inflammatory bowel disease, hemorrhoids, and diverticulitis.[6]

Whole grains can be used as breakfast cereals, side dishes, casseroles, or as part of the main entree.

Breads, Cereals, and Starchy Vegetables
One of the following equals one exchange:

Breads
Bagel, small, ½
Dinner roll, 1
Dried bread crumbs, 3 tbsp
English muffin, small, ½

Tortilla (6-inch diameter), 1
Whole wheat, rye, or pumpernickel, 1 slice

Cereals
Bran flakes, ½ cup
Cornmeal (dry), 2 tbsp
Cereal (cooked), ½ cup
Flour, 2½ tbsp
Grits (cooked), ½ cup
Pasta (cooked), ½ cup
Puffed cereal (unsweetened), 1 cup
Rice or barley (cooked), ½ cup
Wheat germ, ¼ cup
Other unsweetened cereal, ¾ cup

Crackers
Arrowroot, 3
Graham (2½-inch square), 2
Matzo (4 × 6 inches), ½
Rye wafers (2 × 3½ inches), 3
Saltines, 6

Starchy vegetables
Corn kernels, ⅓ cup
Corn on cob, 1 small
Parsnips, ⅔ cup
Potato, mashed, ½ cup
Potato, baked, 1 small
Squash, winter, ½ cup
Yam or sweet potato, ¼ cup

Prepared foods

Biscuit, 2-inch diameter (omit 1 fat exchange), 1

Corn bread, 2 × 2 × 1 inch (omit 1 fat exchange), 1

French fries, 2 to 3 inches long (omit 1 fat exchange), 8

Muffin, small (omit 1 fat exchange), 1

Potato or corn chips (omit 2 fat exchanges), 15

Pancake, 5 × ½ inch (omit 1 fat exchange), 1

Waffle, 5 × ½ inch (omit 1 fat exchange), 1

Legumes

Legumes (beans) are among the oldest cultivated plants. Fossil records demonstrate that even prehistoric people domesticated and cultivated certain legumes for food. Today, the legumes are a mainstay of most diets worldwide. Legumes are second only to grains in supplying calories and protein to the world's population. Compared to grains, they supply about the same number of total calories, but usually provide two to four times as much protein.

Legumes are often called "the poor people's meat," however, they might be better known as the "healthy people's meat." Although lacking some key amino acids, when legumes are combined with grains they form what is known as a complete protein.

Legumes are fantastic foods, rich in important nutrients and health-promoting compounds. Legumes help improve liver function and lower cholesterol levels, and they are extremely effective in improving blood sugar control.

Legumes and Flatulence   One of the problems associated with legumes is increased intestinal flatulence (gas) or intestinal discomfort. Most humans pass gas a total of 14 times per day for a total of one pint. About half of the gas is swallowed air and another 40% is carbon dioxide given off by the bacteria in the intestines. The remaining 10% is a mixture of hydrogen, methane, and sulfur compounds and byproducts of bacteria such as indoles, skatoles, ammonia, and hydrogen sulfide. It is this last fraction that is responsible for the offensive odors.

The flatulence-causing compounds in legumes are primarily oligosaccharides, which are composed of three to five sugar molecules linked together in such a way that the body cannot digest or absorb them. Because the body cannot absorb or digest these oligosaccharides, they pass into the intestines where bacteria break them down. Gas is produced by the bacteria as they digest the oligosaccharides. Navy and lima beans are generally the most offensive, while peanuts are the least because of the lower level of these compounds.

The amount of oligosaccharides in legumes and thus the amount of flatulence produced by them can be significantly reduced by properly cooking or sprouting legumes. A commercial enzyme preparation (Beano) is also available to help reduce flatulence.

Cooking Dried Legumes   Although most legumes can be purchased precooked in cans, cooking your own offers significant economic as well as health benefits due to less salt and the higher nutrient value of home-cooked beans.

Dried legumes are best prepared by first soaking them overnight in an appropriate amount of water (see below). This is best done in the refrigerator to prevent fermentation. Soaking will usually cut the cooking time dramatically. If soaking overnight is not possible, here is an alternate method: Place the dried legumes in an appropriate amount of water in a pot. For each cup of dried legumes, add ¼ teaspoon of baking soda, bring to a boil for at least 2 minutes and then set aside to soak for at least an hour. The baking soda will soften the legumes

Table 8.1   Guide for Cooking Legumes

(1 cup dry)	Water	Cooking Time (if presoaked)	Yield
Black beans	4 cups	1½ hours	2 cups
Black-eyed peas	3 cups	1 hour	2 cups
Chickpeas	4 cups	2½–3 hours	2–3 cups
Kidney beans	3 cups	1½ hours	2 cups
Lentil or split peas	3 cups	½–1 hour	2 cups
Lima beans	2 cups	1½ hours	2 cups
Navy beans	3 cups	1–1½ hours	2 cups
Pinto beans	3 cups	2–2½ hours	2–3 cups
Soybeans	4 cups	3 hours	2 cups

and help break down the troublesome oligosaccharides. The baking soda will also help to reduce the amount of cooking time. After soaking, beans should be simmered with a minimum of stirring to keep them firm and unbroken. A pressure cooker or crock pot can also be used for convenience.

Sprouting Legumes   Since legumes are actually seeds, they can be sprouted. Sprouting is thought to not only increase the nutritional value for many of these foods, it is thought to improve digestibility as well. Many sprouts (such as alfalfa, mung bean, garbanzo beans, and lentils) are available at grocery stores. Alfalfa sprouts are, by far, the most popular.

Sprouting at home is quite easy for most nuts, seeds, grains, and legumes. All you need is a large glass jar or, better yet, invest in a sprouting jar with different types of lids. After rinsing, place the item to be sprouted in the jar and cover with water for 24 hours. You may need to rinse the item once or twice and re-cover with water. After the initial 24 hours, pour out the water, rinse, and allow the moist sprouts to sit in an area without direct sunlight. Rinse the sprouts twice daily. Once the item has sprouted (usually one to two days) it can be placed in more direct sunlight if desired. Most sprouts will be ready to eat in a day or two after they have sprouted.

Legumes
One-half cup of the following cooked or sprouted beans equals one exchange:

Black-eyed peas

Garbanzo beans (chickpeas)

Kidney beans

Lentils

Lima beans

Pinto beans

Soybeans, including tofu (omit 1 fat exchange)

Split peas

Other dried beans and peas

Fats and Oils

Saturated fats are known to exert negative effects on glucose control and are linked to both diabetes and hypoglycemia. Saturated fats are typically animal fats and are solid at room temperature. In contrast, vegetable fats are liquid at room temperature and are referred to as unsaturated fats or oils. The human body requires certain oils. Specifically, our bodies require the fatty acids linoleic and linolenic acid. These fatty acids function in our bodies as components of nerve cells, cellular membranes, and hormonelike substances known as prostaglandins. Increased consumption of essential fatty acids has been shown to lower cholesterol levels and improve many aspects of diabetes.

While essential fatty acids are critical to human health, too much fat in the diet, especially saturated fat, is linked to numerous cancers, heart disease, and strokes. It is strongly recommended by most nutritional experts that your total fat intake be kept below 30% of the total calories. It is also recommended that at least twice as much unsaturated fats be consumed as saturated fats. This recommendation is easy to follow by simply reducing the amount of animal products in your diet, increasing the amount of nuts and seeds consumed, and using natural polyunsaturated oils.

Most commercially available salad dressings, as well as those in restaurants, are full of the wrong type of fats and oils. Salad dressings are the perfect opportunity to use some of the more polyunsaturated and therapeutic vegetable oils such as flaxseed, safflower, sunflower, and soy. Here is an example:

Basil Dressing

Makes 6 servings (2 tablespoons per serving)

¼ cup flaxseed oil
3 tablespoons fresh lemon juice
¼ cup water
2 tablespoons minced fresh basil or 1½ teaspoons dried basil
1 teaspoon finely chopped garlic
Black pepper to taste

Combine all ingredients in a blender or food processor and mix thoroughly.

In addition to saturated fats, margarine should also be avoided. During the process of margarine and shortening manufacture, vegetable oils are *hydrogenated,* which means that a hydrogen molecule is added to the natural unsaturated fatty acid molecules of the vegetable oil in order to make it more saturated (solid). Hydrogenation, the adding of hydrogen molecules, results in changing the structure of the natural fatty acid to many unnatural fatty acid forms.

Many researchers and nutritionists have been concerned about the health effects of margarine and shortening since they were first introduced. Although many Americans assume they are doing their body good by consuming margarine instead of butter and other saturated fats, in truth they are actually doing *more* harm. Margarine and other hydrogenated vegetable oils not only raise LDL cholesterol, they also lower the protective HDL cholesterol level, interfere with essential fatty acid metabolism, and are suspected of being causes of certain cancers.[7] If you desire a butter-like spread, non-hydrogenated canola oil products such as Spectrum from Spectrum Naturals are available in health food stores.

Fats and Oils
Each of the following equals one exchange:

> *Polyunsaturated*
> Vegetable Oils
> > Canola, 1 tsp
> > Corn, 1 tsp
> > Flaxseed, 1 tsp
> > Safflower, 1 tsp
> > Soy, 1 tsp
> > Sunflower, 1 tsp
> > Avocado (4-inch diameter), ⅛
> > Almonds, 10 whole

Pecans, 2 large
Peanuts:
    Spanish, 20 whole
    Virginia, 10 whole
Walnuts, 6 small
Seeds
    Flax, 1 tbsp
    Pumpkin, 1 tbsp
    Sesame, 1 tbsp
    Sunflower, 1 tbsp

Monounsaturated
Olive oil, 1 tsp
Olives, 5 small

Saturated (use sparingly)
Butter, 1 tsp
Bacon, 1 slice
Cream, light or sour, 2 tbsp
Cream, heavy, 1 tbsp
Cream cheese, 1 tbsp
Salad dressings, 2 tsp
Mayonnaise, 1 tsp

Milk

Is milk for "everybody"? Definitely not. Many people are allergic to milk or lack the enzymes necessary to digest milk. The drinking of cow's milk is a relatively new dietary practice for humans. This may be the reason so many people have difficulty with milk. Furthermore, there is evidence that early exposure to cow's milk in infants is a trigger not only for food allergies but also for developing type I diabetes.[8] Several studies have shown that the consumption of milk is directly related to the development of type I diabetes. Certainly milk consumption should be avoided in all children under one year of age.

Another reason to avoid milk is that a milk protein known as *casein* appears to promote atherosclerosis.[9] Many meal-replacement formulas, including Ultra SlimFast, contain casein. Casein is also used in glues, molded plastics, and paints. Good alternatives to milk and casein-containing formulas are soy milk or soy-based formulas. Unlike casein, soy protein actually lowers cholesterol levels.[10]

Milk consumption in older children and adults should be limited to no more than one or two servings per day. Choose nonfat products.

Milk and Milk Products
One cup equals one exchange.

Nonfat milk or yogurt

2% milk (omit 1 fat exchange)

Lowfat yogurt (omit 1 fat exchange)

Whole milk (omit 2 fat exchanges)

Whole milk yogurt (omit 2 fat exchanges)

Meats, Fish, Cheese, and Eggs

When choosing from this category, it is important to choose primarily from the lowfat group and remove the skin of poultry. This will keep the amount of saturated fat low. Although many people advocate vegetarianism, the exchange list below provides high concentrations of certain nutrients difficult to get in an entirely vegetarian diet, such as the full-range of amino acids, vitamin B_{12}, and iron. Use these foods in small amounts as "condiments" in the diet rather than as mainstays. Definitely stay away from cured meats such as bacon, pastrami, and ham; these foods are rich in compounds that can lead to the formation of cancer-causing compounds known as nitrosamines. A possible exception to the recommendation of *reducing* your intake of animal foods are cold-water fish such as salmon, mackerel, and herring, which provide oils known as omega-3 fatty acids. These beneficial oils have been shown in hundreds of studies to lower cholesterol and triglyceride levels, thereby reducing the risk of heart disease and strokes. The omega-3 fatty acids are also being recommended to treat high blood pressure, other cardiovascular diseases, cancer, auto-immune diseases such as multiple sclerosis and rheumatoid arthritis, allergies and inflammation, eczema, psoriasis, and many other diseases.[11]

Meats, Fish, Cheese, and Eggs
Each of the following equals one exchange:

Lowfat (less than 15% fat content)
Beef, 1 oz
> Baby beef, chipped beef, chuck, steak (flank, plate), tenderloin plate ribs, round (bottom, top), all cuts rump, spare ribs, tripe

Cottage cheese, lowfat, ¼ cup

Fish, 1 oz

Lamb, 1 oz
> Leg, rib, sirloin, loin (roast and chops), shank, shoulder

Poultry (chicken or turkey without skin), 1 oz

Veal, 1 oz
> Leg, loin, rib, shank, shoulder, cutlet

Medium fat (for each omit ½ fat exchange)

Beef, 1 oz

  Ground (15% fat), canned corned beef, rib eye, round (ground commercial)

Cheese, 1 oz

  Mozzarella, ricotta, farmer's, Parmesan

Eggs, 1

Organ meats, 1 oz

Peanut butter, 2 tbsp

Pork, 1 oz

  Loin (all tenderloin), picnic and boiled ham, shoulder, Boston butt, Canadian bacon

High fat (for each exchange omit 1 fat exchange)

Beef, 1 oz

  Brisket, corned beef, ground beef (more than 20% fat), hamburger, roasts (rib), steaks (club and rib)

Cheese, cheddar, 1 oz

Duck or goose, 1 oz

Lamb breast, 1 oz

Pork, 1 oz

  Spareribs, ground pork, country-style ham, deviled ham

Menu Planning

The Healthy Exchange System was created to ensure that you are consuming a healthful diet that is providing adequate levels of nutrients in their proper ratio. It is important that you have determined your caloric needs and have calculated the number of servings required from each Healthy Exchange List. This will help a great deal when constructing a daily menu.

Breakfast

Breakfast is an absolute must. Healthful breakfast choices include whole grain cereals, muffins, and breads along with fresh whole fruit or fresh fruit juice. Cereals, both hot and cold, and preferably from whole grains, may be the best food choices for breakfast. The complex carbohydrates in the grains provide sustained energy and an evaluation of data from the National Health and Nutrition Examination Survey II (a national survey of the nutritional and health practices of Americans) disclosed that serum cholesterol levels are lowest among adults eating whole grain cereal for breakfast.[12] Although those individuals who consumed other breakfast foods had higher blood cholesterol levels, levels were highest among those who typically skipped breakfast.

Lunch

Lunch is a great time to enjoy a healthful bowl of soup, a large salad, and some whole grain bread. Bean soups and other legume dishes are especially good lunch selections for people with diabetes and blood sugar problems due to their ability to improve blood sugar regulation. Legumes are filling yet low in calories.

Dinner

For dinner, the most healthful meals contain a fresh vegetable salad, a cooked vegetable side dish or soup, whole grains, and legumes. The whole grains may be provided in bread, pasta, pizza, as a side dish, or as part of an entree. The legumes can be utilized in soups, salads, and main dishes.

Although a varied diet rich in whole grains, vegetables, and legumes provides optimal levels of protein, some people like to eat meat. The important thing is not to over-consume animal products. Limit your intake to no more than 4 to 6 ounces per day and choose fish, skinless poultry, and lean cuts rather than fat-laden choices.

Final Comments

Just as important as what you eat is how you eat. Here are some simple recommendations to improve digestion:

1. Take time to plan out your meals ahead of time.
2. Eat in a relaxed, quiet environment where your focus is on the food and the people you are enjoying it with.
3. Avoid eating in front of the television.
4. Bless and give thanks for the meal—many others are less fortunate.
5. Eat at a slow to moderate pace.
6. Chew thoroughly. (Although it is often recommended to chew food 100 times before swallowing, in my opinion this is a bit much. just be sure that the food is chewed thoroughly and well-mixed with saliva.)
7. Avoid swallowing too much air.
8. Drink water with your meal only if necessary and never drink ice water. Water may dilute the concentration of digestive factors in the stomach and ice water may lead to reduction of blood supply to the stomach.
9. Take time to relax (if possible) after a meal in order to let your digestive system go to work.
10. Visualize your body digesting and assimilating the meal.

8

Inflammatory Bowel Disease

Inflammatory bowel disease (IBD) is a general term for a group of chronic inflammatory disorders of the bowel. It is divided into two major categories: Crohn's disease and ulcerative colitis. Clinically, IBD is characterized by recurrent inflammation of specific intestinal segments resulting in diverse symptoms.

Crohn's Disease

Crohn's disease is characterized by an inflammatory reaction throughout the entire thickness of the bowel wall. In approximately 40% of cases, however, the inflammatory lesions (granulomas) are either poorly developed or totally absent. The original description in 1932 by Crohn and colleagues localized the disease to segments in the ileum, the terminal portion of the small intestine. However, the same granulomatous process may involve the mucosa of the mouth, esophagus, stomach, duodenum, jejunum, and colon.

Crohn's disease of the small intestine is also known as *regional enteritis,* while involvement of the colon is known as Crohn's disease of the colon or *granulomatous colitis.*

Crohn's Disease Diagnostic Summary
> Intermittent bouts of diarrhea, low-grade fever, and right lower quadrant pain
>
> Loss of appetite, weight loss, flatulence, and malaise
>
> Abdominal tenderness, especially in the right lower quadrant, with signs of peritoneal irritation and an abdominal or pelvic mass
>
> X-rays show abnormality of the terminal ileum

Ulcerative Colitis

In ulcerative colitis, there is a nonspecific inflammatory response limited largely to the lining of the colon. Crohn's disease and ulcerative colitis do share many common features and, where appropriate, will be discussed together. Otherwise they will be discussed as separate entities.

Ulcerative Colitis Diagnostic Summary
> Bloody diarrhea with cramps in the lower abdomen
>
> Mild abdominal tenderness, weight loss, and fever
>
> Rectal examination may show perianal irritation, fissures, hemorrhoids, fistulas, and abscesses
>
> Diagnosis confirmed by x-ray and sigmoidoscopy

Common Features Shared by Crohn's Disease and Ulcerative Colitis

> 1. The colon is frequently involved in Crohn's disease and is invariably involved in ulcerative colitis.

2. Although rare, patients with ulcerative colitis who have total colon involvement may develop a so-called *backwash ileitis.* Thus, both Crohn's disease and ulcerative colitis may cause changes in the small intestine.

3. Patients with Crohn's disease often have close relatives with ulcerative colitis, and vice versa.

4. When there is no granulomatous reaction in Crohn's disease of the colon, the two lesions may resemble each other, both in the clinical picture and the biopsy result.

5. The many epidemiological similarities between the two diseases include age, race, sex, and geographic distribution.

6. Both conditions are associated with similar extraintestinal manifestations.

7. The causative factors appear to be parallel for the two conditions.

8. Both conditions are associated with an increased frequency of colonic carcinoma.

The rates of the two diseases differ slightly, with most studies showing ulcerative colitis to be more common than Crohn's disease. The current estimate of the yearly rate of newly diagnosed cases of ulcerative colitis in western Europe and the United States is approximately 6 to 8 cases per 100,000, and the estimated rate of the total number of cases is approximately 70 to 150 cases per 100,000. The estimate for the yearly rate of newly diagnosed cases of Crohn's disease is approximately 2 cases per 100,000, while the total number of cases is estimated at 20 to 40 per 100,000. The rate of Crohn's disease is increasing in Western cultures.

Inflammatory bowel disease (IBD) may occur at any age, but most often it occurs between the ages of 15 and

35. Females are affected slightly more often than males. Caucasians develop the disease two to five times more often than those of African or Asian descent, while Jews have a three- to sixfold higher incidence compared with non-Jews.

Theories about the cause of IBD can be divided into several groups:

1. Genetic predisposition
2. Infectious agent or agents
3. Immunologic abnormality
4. Dietary factors
5. An assortment of miscellaneous concepts implicating psychosomatic, vascular, traumatic, and other mechanisms

Genetic Predisposition

Although the search for a specific genetic marker for IBD has been futile, several factors suggest a genetic predisposition. As already mentioned, IBD is two to four times more common in Caucasians than non-Caucasians, and three to six times more common in Jews than non-Jews. In addition, in 15% to 40% of the cases, multiple members of a family have Crohn's disease or ulcerative colitis.

Infectious Agents

Many microorganisms have been hailed as potential causes of IBD, but the idea that a microbial agent is responsible for IBD is still a hotly debated subject. Viruses—such as rotavirus, Epstein-Barr virus, and cytomegalovirus—and mycobacteria continue to be favored candidates. Other candidates include Pseudomonas-like organisms, chlamydia, and *Yersinia enterocolitica*.

Immunologic Abnormality

An overwhelming amount of evidence points to immune-system disturbances in IBD, but whether these disturbances are causal or secondary phenomena remains unclear. Theories linking immune-system derangements as causes of IBD have been proposed, but the current evidence seems to indicate that these derangements are probably secondary to the disease process.

Dietary Factors

Despite the fact that a dietary cause of Crohn's disease is hardly considered (if mentioned at all) in most standard medical and gastroenterology texts, several lines of evidence strongly support dietary factors as being the most important causative factor.[1-13]

The incidence of Crohn's disease is increasing in cultures consuming a Western diet (high in saturated fats, refined carbohydrates, and sugar) while it is virtually nonexistent in cultures consuming a more "primitive" diet (one that is high in fiber).[1-5] Because food is the major factor in determining the intestinal environment, the considerable change in dietary habits over the last century could explain the rising rates of Crohn's disease.

Several studies that analyzed the pre-illness diet of patients with Crohn's disease have found that people who develop Crohn's disease habitually eat more refined sugar and less raw fruit and vegetables and dietary fiber than healthy people.[1-5] In one study, the pre-illness intake of refined sugar in Crohn's disease patients was nearly twice that of controls (122 g per day versus 65 g per day).[5] One researcher found that before the onset of disease, Crohn's disease patients had eaten corn flakes more frequently than controls.[14] Although other researchers could not verify this specific finding, corn flakes are high in refined carbohydrates and are derived from a very common allergen (corn).

Much of the controversy over the role of pre-illness diet in the etiology of Crohn's disease is largely due to the fact that the only way to assess diet is from post-diagnostic interviews. Studies where the interview has taken place within the first six months of diagnosis tend to be more supportive than studies done more than seven months after diagnosis. In contrast, patients with ulcerative colitis do not show an increased consumption of refined carbohydrates when compared with controls.[15]

Another important dietary factor that is entirely overlooked in the standard medical texts is the role of food allergy. Support for this hypothesis is offered in clinical studies that have utilized an elemental diet, total parenteral nutrition, or an exclusion diet with great success in the treatment of IBD.[7-13] These restricted diets and the roles of food allergy and dietary fiber are discussed in greater detail below.

Miscellaneous Factors in IBD

Psychosomatic factors, vascular disturbances, and chronic trauma have received consideration in the origin of IBD, but at present are not considered significant mechanisms. While there is little evidence directly relating psychological factors to the initiation of IBD, there is little doubt that emotional factors are important in modifying the course of the disease.

The Natural History of Crohn's Disease

Little is known concerning the natural course of Crohn's disease because virtually all patients with the disease undergo standard medical care (drugs and/or surgery) or alternative therapy. The only exceptions are those patients in clinical trials who are assigned to the placebo group.[16–18] Even these patients do not represent the natural course of the disease, since they are frequently seen by physicians and other members of a health care team and are taking medication, even if it is only in the form of a placebo. However, if proper evaluation of therapies for IBD is to occur, there must be a greater understanding of its natural history.

This understanding is particularly important for alternative practitioners, because it is commonly believed that standard medical care often interferes with the normal efforts of the body to restore itself to health. However, administration of corticosteroids, hospitalization, and even surgical heroic measures do have their place in many instances and should be used when appropriate.

Researchers in the National Cooperative Crohn's Disease Study (NCCDS) reviewed 77 patients who received placebo therapy in part 1 of the 17-week study.[16,17] They all had active disease, as defined by a Crohn's disease activity index (CDAI) of above 150. Of the patients completing the study, no patient died; only 7 (9%) suffered a major worsening of their disease (i.e., either they developed a major fistula or required abdominal surgery); 25 (32%) suffered a lesser worsening (increase in the CDAI to >450 or presence of a fever of at least 100 degrees Fahrenheit for two weeks); 25 (32%) were considered failures, because their CDAI remained >150; and 20 patients (26%) achieved clinical remission. On at least one occasion during the 17 weeks of therapy, 49% of the patients were found to have a CDAI of <150.

The patients who responded favorably to the placebo continued to be observed on placebo therapy for up to two years (part 1, phase 2). While none of these patients' x-rays worsened during phase 1 or phase 2, 18% actually showed improvement on their intestinal x-rays. Of the patients responding to the placebo, the majority (70%) remained in remission at one year, and a fair number

(45%) remained in remission at two years. These results indicate that many patients will undergo spontaneous remission, approximately 20% at one year and 12% at two years. However, when another factor is considered, the success of the placebo therapy rises dramatically. In patients having no previous history of steroid therapy, 41% achieved remission after 17 weeks. In addition, 23% of this group continued in remission after two years, compared to only 4% of the group with a prior history of steroid use.

The European Cooperative Crohn's Disease Study (ECCDS), although different in some details of method, was quite similar to the NCCDS.[16,18] In the ECCDS, 110 patients (68 patients with prior treatment and 42 patients with no prior treatment) constituted the placebo group. The results of the study indicated that 55% of the total placebo group achieved remission by 100 days, 34% remained in remission at 300 days, and 21% remained in remission at 700 days. Like the NCCDS, the ECCDS demonstrated that patients with no prior therapy have an increased likelihood of remission.

While one group of researchers did not advocate placebo therapy, they did carefully point out that once remission is achieved, 75% of the patients will continue in remission at the end of one year and up to 63% at the end of two years, regardless of the maintenance therapy used. These results suggest that the key is achieving remission, which, once attained, can be maintained by conservative nondrug therapy rather than the "medicines we are currently using with their limited efficacy and known toxicity."[16]

Abnormalities Found in Inflammatory Bowel Disease

Prostaglandin Metabolism

Prostaglandins are hormonelike substances manufactured from essential fatty acids that govern many bodily functions including inflammation. Prostaglandin levels are greatly increased in the colonic mucosa, serum, and stools of patients with IBD. Specifically, these patients show an increase in the synthesis of inflammatory compounds known as leukotrienes.[19-22] These compounds are produced by neutrophils and are known to amplify the inflammatory process and cause intestinal cramping and pain.

To reduce the formation of these inflammatory compounds, reduce or eliminate your consumption of meat and dairy products while increasing your consumption of omega-3 fatty acids by increasing your intake of cold-water fish (such as salmon, mackerel, herring, and halibut). These fish are good sources of the longer chain omega-3 fatty acids—eicosapentaenoic acid (EPA) and docosahexanoic acid (DHA). It is also a good idea to take one tablespoon of flaxseed oil each day. Flaxseed oil contains alpha-linolenic acid, the essential omega-3 fatty acid, which the body can convert to EPA.

Mucin Defects

Mucins are glycoproteins (proteins with sugar molecules attached) that are largely responsible for the viscous and elastic characteristics of secreted mucus. Alterations in mucin composition and content in the colonic mucosa have been reported in patients with ulcerative colitis.[23-25] The factors responsible for this appear to be a dramatic decrease in the mucus content of the mucus-producing (goblet) cells (proportional to the severity of the disease) as well as a decrease in the major sulfur-containing mucin.

In contrast, these abnormalities are not found in patients with Crohn's disease. It is significant that while the mucin content of the goblet cells returns to normal during remission of ulcerative colitis, the sulfur-containing mucin deficiency does not. The specific components of the sulfur-containing mucin and the cause of its lower concentration have not yet been determined. These mucin abnormalities are also thought to be a major factor in the increased risk of colon cancer in these patients.

Many of the herbs used historically in the treatment of ulcerative colitis are demulcents (agents that soothe irritated mucous membranes and promote the secretion of mucus). This effect of demulcents appears to be very helpful and supports the use of demulcents such as DGL, marshmallow root, and slippery elm in ulcerative colitis.

Intestinal Microflora

The fecal flora of patients with Crohn's disease has been found to be greatly disturbed.[26] Indications are that these alterations in fecal flora are *not* secondary to the disease. Alterations in the *metabolic activity* of the various bacteria are thought to be more important than alterations in the *number* of bacteria per se. In addition, it is thought that specific bacterial cell components (which vary even within the same species) are responsible for promoting destruction of the intestinal cells.

Carrageenan   Researchers investigating IBD often use carrageenan (a compound extracted from red seaweeds) to experimentally induce the disease in animals. In the initial experiments reported by Marcus and Watt in 1969, 1% and 5% carrageenan solutions were provided as the exclusive source of oral fluids for guinea pigs.[27] Over a period of several days the animals lost weight, developed anemia, had bloody diarrhea, and developed ulcerative colitis. These results have since been confirmed by numerous investigators and in studies involving other animal species, including primates.[26-30]

In its natural state this polymer has a molecular weight of 100,000 to 800,000, but in the studies it was degraded by mild acidic hydrolysis to yield products with weights in the vicinity of 30,000. These smaller molecules are thought to be responsible for inducing the ulcerative damage in the animal studies. Carrageenan compounds are used by the food industry as stabilizing and suspending agents, with different molecular weight polymers being used for a variety of purposes. Typically, carrageenans used in the food industry have a molecular weight greater than 100,000. Carrageenan is widely used in milk and chocolate milk products (ice cream, cottage cheese, milk chocolate, etc.) due to its ability to stabilize milk proteins.

As suggestive as the animal studies are in linking ulcerative colitis with carrageenan, no lesions of IBD were observed in healthy human subjects fed enormous quantities of degraded carrageenan.[31] However, differences in intestinal bacterial flora are probably responsible for this discrepancy, as germ-free animals do not display carrageenan-induced damage either.

The bacteria that has been linked to facilitating the carrageenan-induced damage in animals is a strain of *Bacteroides vulgatus*.[26] This organism is found in much higher concentrations (six times as high) in the fecal cultures of patients with Crohn's disease. When the data is evaluated, it implies that while carrageenan can be metabolized into non-damaging components in most human subjects, those individuals with an overgrowth of *Bacteroides vulgatus* may be at risk. Strict avoidance of carrageenan appears warranted at this time for individuals with IBD until further research clarifies its safety for these patients. If you have IBD, read food labels carefully.

Extra-Gastrointestinal Manifestations

Over 100 disorders, known as *extraintestinal lesions* (EIL), constitute a diverse group of systemic complications of

IBD.[32] The most common EIL in adults is arthritis, which is found in about 25% of patients. Two types are typically described, the more common being peripheral arthritis affecting the knees, ankles, and wrists. Arthritis is more frequently found in patients with colon involvement. Severity of symptoms is typically proportional to disease activity. Less frequently, the arthritis affects the spine. Symptoms are low back pain and stiffness with eventual limitation of motion. This EIL occurs predominantly in males and is fairly indistinguishable from typical ankylosing spondylitis (rheumatoid arthritis of the spine). In fact, it may precede the bowel symptoms by several years. There is probably a consistent underlying factor in both the progression of ankylosing spondylitis and IBD.

Skin manifestations are also common, being seen in approximately 15% of patients. The skin lesions can be quite severe, including gangrene and/or painful, red lumps (e.g., erythema nodosum and pyoderma gangrenosum), but are usually simply annoying like canker sores. In fact, recurrent canker sores occur in approximately 10% of patients with IBD.[32]

Serious liver disease (i.e., sclerosing cholangitis, chronic active hepatitis, cirrhosis, etc.) also is a common EIL, affecting 3% to 7% of people with IBD. If individuals are demonstrating liver enzyme abnormalities, they should take silymarin—a group of flavonoid compounds derived from milk thistle (*Silybum marianum*). These compounds exert tremendous effect on protecting the liver from damage as well as enhancing detoxification processes.[33] Silymarin products are available at health food stores. The standard dosage for silymarin is 70 to 210 mg, three times daily.

Other common EIL are inflammation of blood vessels, impaired blood flow to the fingers or toes, inflammatory eye manifestations (episcleritis, iritis, and uveitis), kidney stones, gallstones, and in children, failure to grow, thrive, and mature normally.

IBD's Effects on General Nutrition

Many nutritional complications occur during the course of IBD.[34-36] Because these can have a significant influence on the well-being, and perhaps also the mortality, of those with IBD, every effort should be made to ensure optimal nutritional status. The major mechanisms that contribute to nutritional depletion in these patients are listed below:

Causes of Malnutrition in Inflammatory Bowel Disease

Decreased food intake

Disease-induced (pain, diarrhea, nausea, anorexia)

Doctor-induced (restrictive diets without supplementation)

Malabsorption

Decreased absorptive surface due to disease or surgical resection (removal of diseased segments by surgery)

Bile salt deficiency after surgical resection

Bacterial overgrowth

Drugs (e.g., corticosteroids, sulfasalazine, cholestyramine)

Increased secretion and nutrient loss

Protein-losing enteropathy (loss of protein due to shedding of intestinal cells)

Electrolyte, mineral, and trace mineral loss in diarrhea

Increased utilization and requirements for nutrients

Inflammation, fever, infection

Increased intestinal cell turnover

A decreased food intake is the most important mechanism of nutritional deficiency in the patients with IBD, and deficient calorie intake is the most common nutritional deficit in patients requiring hospitalization. Often the patient feels significant pain, diarrhea, nausea, and/or other symptoms after a meal, resulting in a subtle diminution in dietary intake. Weight loss is prevalent in 65% to 75% of IBD patients.[34]

Malabsorption can be anticipated in patients with extensive involvement of the small intestine and in patients who have had surgical resection of segments of the small intestine. Particularly common is fat malabsorption, resulting in significant caloric loss as well as loss of fat-soluble vitamins and minerals. Involvement of the ileum or resection of that area typically results in bile acid malabsorption. Because of the laxative effect of bile acids on the colon, this may result in a chronic watery diarrhea. Electrolyte and trace mineral deficiency should be suspected in patients with a history of chronic diarrhea, while calcium and magnesium deficiency may be a result of chronic fat malabsorption (steatorrhea).

Increased secretion and nutrient loss due to the exudative and inflammatory nature of IBD often occur. In particular, there is a significant loss of plasma proteins across the damaged and inflamed mucosa. The loss of protein may exceed the ability of the liver to replace plasma proteins, despite a high protein intake. The chronic loss of blood often leads to iron depletion and anemia.

The most common drugs used in the allopathic treatment of IBD are corticosteroids (e.g., prednisone) and sulfasalazine, both of which increase nutritional needs. Corticosteroids are known to stimulate protein catabolism; depress protein synthesis; decrease the absorption of calcium and phosphorus; increase the urinary excretion of vitamin C, calcium, potassium, and zinc; increase blood glucose, serum triglycerides, and serum cholesterol; increase the requirements for vitamin B_6, ascorbic acid, folate, and vitamin D; decrease bone formation; and impair wound healing. Sulfasalazine inhibits the absorption and transport of folate; decreases serum folate and iron; and increases the urinary excretion of ascorbic acid. The last consideration in the causes of nutrient deficiency in IBD is the nutritional consequences of a chronic inflammatory and/or infectious disease. This topic has not been fully investigated, and the only conclusion that currently can be made is that protein requirements may be increased in patients with acute worsening of IBD. Typically, patients with IBD require perhaps as much as 25% more protein than the usual recommended allowance.[34-36]

Correcting Nutritional Deficiencies

The importance of correcting nutritional deficiencies in patients with IBD cannot be overstated. Nutrient deficiencies, both macro and micro, lead to altered gastrointestinal function and structure, which may result in the patient entering a vicious cycle. That is, the secondary effects of malnutrition on the gastrointestinal tract may lead to a further increase in malabsorption, further decreasing nutrient status.

Foremost in nutritional therapy is providing adequate caloric intake. The first step in dietary treatment involves the use of either an elemental or an elimination diet.

Elemental Diets

The elemental diet has been shown to be an effective nontoxic alternative to corticosteroids as the primary treatment of acute IBD.[7-10] An elemental diet is one that is purported to contain all essential nutrients, with protein being provided only in the form of predigested or free-form amino acids. The improvements noted on an elemental diet are, however, probably not primarily related to nutritional improvement. Although the improvement could be a result of alterations in the fecal flora (which have been noted to occur in patients consuming an elemental diet), a stronger case could be made for a secondary immune mechanism being bypassed during elemental feeding; in other words, the elemental diet is serving as an allergy elimination diet.

Hospitalization is often required for satisfactory administration of elemental diets. Relapse is quite common when patients resume normal eating. An elimination diet, may be a more acceptable alternative in the treatment of IBD, particularly when treating chronic IBD.

Elimination (Oligoantigenic) Diets

Although food allergy has long been considered an important causative factor in the development of IBD, studies have only recently utilized an elimination diet in the treatment of IBD.[11-13] (Elimination diets are described in detail on page 106). These studies demonstrate that an elimination diet should be the primary therapy in the treatment of chronic IBD. The most common offending foods were found to be wheat and dairy products. The typical response to an elimination diet is clinical remission.

An alternative approach is to determine the actual allergens by laboratory methods, preferably a method that measures both IgG- and IgE-mediated reactions. The allergens are then either avoided, or a rotary diversified diet is used if it is appropriate (see page 110).

High Complex-Carbohydrate, High-Fiber Diet

Treatment with a high-fiber diet has been shown to have a favorable effect on the course of Crohn's disease.[6] This is in direct contrast to one of the oldest allopathic dietary treatments of IBD—a low-fiber diet. Although some foods,

Table 8.1 Prevalence of Nutritional Deficiency in Patients with Inflammatory Bowel Disease[34]

Deficiency	Prevalence (%)
Iron deficiency	40
Low serum vitamin B_{12}	48
Low serum folate	54–64
Low serum magnesium	14–33
Low serum potassium	6–20
Low serum retinol	21
Low serum ascorbate	12
Low serum 25-OH-vitamin D	25–65
Low serum zinc	40–50

such as wheat bran, may be too "rough" to handle, the dietary treatment of IBD should utilize an unrefined carbohydrate, fiber-rich diet combined with an avoidance or rotary diversified diet. This latter combination is much more effective than just a high-fiber diet alone.[12]

Dietary fiber has a profound effect on the intestinal environment and is thought to promote a more optimal intestinal flora composition.[37] However, considering the high degree of intolerance to wheat found in patients with IBD, and the known roughness of wheat bran, supplemental wheat bran is not the fiber of choice for these patients.

Take a High-Quality Multiple Vitamin and Mineral Formula

It is absolutely essential that patients with IBD take a high-quality multiple vitamin and mineral supplement providing all of the known vitamins and minerals. Use the recommendations in Table 8.2 to provide an optimum intake range in selecting a high-quality multiple. The majority of individuals with IBD suffer from nutritional deficiencies. In addition to the deficiencies listed in Table 8.1, low levels of vitamin K, copper, niacin, and vitamin E have also been reported.[34]

Take Additional Antioxidants

In addition to taking a high-potency multiple vitamin and mineral formula, patients with IBD will need to take additional antioxidants. The two primary antioxidants in the human body are vitamin C and vitamin E. Vitamin C is an *aqueous phase* antioxidant, which means that it is found in body compartments composed of water. In contrast, vitamin E is a *lipid phase* antioxidant because it is found in fat-soluble body compartments such as cell membranes and fatty molecules. For good antioxidant protection, I would recommend taking the following each day for patients with IBD:

Vitamin E (d-alpha tocopherol)	400 to 800 IU
Vitamin C (ascorbic acid)	1,000 to 3,000 mg

The Role of Zinc, Folic Acid, and Vitamin B_{12} in IBD

Three nutrients deserve special mention in the treatment of IBD—zinc, folic acid, and vitamin B_{12}. Zinc deficiency is a well-known complication of Crohn's disease, due to low dietary intake, poor absorption, and excess fecal losses.[38] Evidence of zinc deficiency occurs in approximately 45% of Crohn's disease patients and for a similar percentage of ulcerative colitis patients. Low zinc concentrations in the blood, low zinc levels in the hair, malabsorption of zinc, altered urinary excretion of zinc, and impaired taste acuity

Table 8.2 Recommended Ranges for Supplemental Vitamins and Minerals

Vitamin	Range for Adults
Vitamin A (retinol)*	5,000 IU

*Women of child-bearing age should not take more than 2,500 IU of retinol daily due to the possible risk of birth defects if becoming pregnant is a possibility.

Vitamin A (from beta-carotene)	5,000–25,000 IU
Vitamin D	100–400 IU
Vitamin E (d-alpha tocopherol)	100–200 IU
Vitamin K (phytonadione)	60–300 mcg
Vitamin C (ascorbic acid)	100–1,000 mg
Vitamin B1 (thiamin)	10–100 mg
Vitamin B2 (riboflavin)	10–50 mg
Niacin	10–100 mg
Niacinamide	10–30 mg
Vitamin B$_6$ (pyridoxine)	25–100 mg
Biotin	100–300 mcg
Pantothenic acid	25–100 mg
Folic acid	400 mcg
Vitamin B$_{12}$	400 mcg
Choline	10–100 mg
Inositol	10–100 mg

Minerals

Boron	1–6 mg
Calcium	250–500 mg
Chromium	200–400 mcg
Copper	1–2 mg
Iodine	50–150 mcg
Iron**	15–30 mg

**Men and postmenopausal women rarely need supplemental iron.

Magnesium	250–500 mg
Manganese	10–15 mg
Molybdenum	10–25 mcg
Potassium	200–500 mg
Selenium	100–200 mcg
Silica	1–25 mg
Vanadium	50–100 mcg
Zinc	15–45 mg

are commonly found in Crohn's disease patients. In addition, many of the complications of the disease may be a direct result of zinc deficiency: poor healing of fissures and fistulas, skin lesions, hypogonadism, growth retardation, retinal dysfunction, depressed immunity, and loss of appetite.

Many patients will not respond to oral or even intravenous zinc supplementation; there appears to be a defect in tissue transport. Intravenous supplementation results in a tremendous increase in urinary zinc excretion, but insignificant clinical results. Several clinical trials using oral zinc sulfate have shown the same lack of results.[39] Supplying zinc in the form of zinc picolinate may be more advantageous, possibly improving both intestinal absorption and tissue transport. Picolinate is a zinc-binding molecule that is secreted by the pancreas and which appears to be better absorbed and utilized than other types of zinc.

Like zinc deficiency, folic acid deficiency also is quite common in IBD, with reports of occurrence ranging from 25% to 64%.[34,40–42] The reason for this deficiency in many cases is the drug sulfasalazine. Correction of folate deficiency is absolutely essential because folate deficiency promotes further malabsorption and diarrhea due to altered structure of the intestinal mucosal cells.[43] These cells have a very rapid turnover (one to four days) and need to have a constant supply of folic acid.

Since vitamin B_{12} is absorbed at the portion of the intestine most commonly affected with Crohn's disease (the terminal ileum), deficiency of this vitamin also is quite common.[34,44] Overall, abnormal B_{12} absorption is found in 48% of patients with Crohn's disease. Often the terminal ileum is surgically removed (resected). If the length of the resection is less than 60 cm, or the extent of the inflammatory lesion is less than 60 cm, adequate absorption may occur. Otherwise, monthly vitamin B_{12} injections (1,000 mcg, intramuscularly) are recommended.

An Old Naturopathic Remedy

Although no research has been done to document its efficacy, an old naturopathic remedy, Robert's Formula, has a long history of use by naturopathic physicians for treating IBD. It is composed of several botanical medicines: *Althea officinalis* (marshmallow root—a demulcent with soothing); *Baptisia tinctora* (wild indigo—used for gastrointestinal infections); *Echinacea angustifolia* (purple coneflower—antibacterial and used to promote normalization of the immune system); *Geranium maculatum* (American cranesbill—used for its astringent action to help heal ulcerations); *Hydrastis canadensis* (goldenseal—inhibits the growth of many disease-causing bacteria); *Symphytum offinale* (comfrey—anti-inflammatory that promotes tissue growth and wound healing); and *Ulmus fulva* (slippery elm—demulcent effect).

Here is a version of the modified Robert's formula you can mix up yourself using powdered herbs available at health food stores:

8 parts *Althea officinalis*

4 parts *Baptisia tinctora*

8 parts *Echinacea angustifolia*

8 parts *Geranium maculatum*

8 parts *Hydrastis canadensis*

8 parts *Ulmus fulva*

8 parts cabbage powder (*Brassica oleracea*)

You can take 1 teaspoon of the above, three times daily. Or you may choose to purchase one of the many commercially available versions. Here is the formulation that I use in my clinical practice (Robert's Complex from Enzymatic Therapy):

Each capsule contains:

Niacinamide, 5 mg

American cranesbill (*Geranium maculatum*), 100 mg

Cabbage (*Brassica oleracea*), 100 mg

Marshmallow extract (8:1) (*Althea officinalis*), 75 mg
(mucilage content 30% to 40%)

Okra (*Hibiscus esculentis*), 75 mg

Slippery elm (*Ulma fulva*), 75 mg

Duodenal substance, 25 mg

Echinacea root extract (*Echinacea angustifolia*), 25 mg
Standardized to contain greater than 3.5%
echinacosides and 0.65% essential oils

Goldenseal extract (*Hydrastis canadensis*), 25 mg
Standardized to contain 8% to 10% total alkaloids
including berberine, hydrastine, and canadine

Pancreatic enzymes, 25 mg

The dosage recommendation is 2 capsules, three times daily.

Crohn's Disease Activity Index (CDAI)

The Crohn's disease activity index was developed as a monitoring tool in the National Cooperative Crohn's Disease Study.[45] It met the basic requirements necessary for the study, i.e., it provided uniform clinical parameters that could be assessed and it produced a consistent numerical index for recording the results of the study. Table 8.3 outlines the variables and formula used to calculate the CDAI.

The CDAI is calculated by adding together eight variables (see Table 8.3). It incorporates both subjective and objective information in determining relative disease activity. When the patient returns with the completed form, the calculation of disease activity can be completed.

Table 8.3 Independent Variables and Formula Used to Calculate the CDAI

X1 Number of liquid or very soft stools in one week.

X2 Sum of seven daily abdominal pain ratings:
0 = none, 1 = mild, 2 = moderate, 3 = severe

X3 Sum of seven daily ratings of general well-being:
0 = well, 1 = slightly below par, 2 = poor, 3 = very poor, 4 = terrible

X4 Symptoms or findings presumed related to Crohn's disease:
1. Arthritis or arthralgia
2. Iritis or uveitis
3. Erythema nodosum, pyoderma gangrenosum, aphthous stomatitis
4. Anal fissure, fistula, or perirectal abscess
5. Other bowel-related fistula
6. Febrile episode > 100 degrees Fahrenheit during past week
(Add 1 for each category corresponding to patient's symptoms.)

X5 Taking Lomotil or opiates for diarrhea:
0 = no, 1 = yes

X6 Abdominal mass:
0 = none, 0.4 = questionable, 1 = present

X7 47 minus hematocrit, males; 42 minus hematocrit, females

X8 100 × (standard weight according to height and weight charts minus body weight)/standard weight

CDAI = 2 multiplied by X1 + 5 multiplied by X2 + 7 multiplied by X3 + 20 multiplied by X4 + 30 multiplied by X5 + 10 multiplied by X6 + 6 multiplied by X7 + X8 multiplied by 8

Generally speaking, CDAI scores below 150 indicate a better prognosis than higher scores. The CDAI is a very useful way to monitor therapeutic progress.

Monitoring of the Pediatric Patient

It is often very difficult to achieve normal growth and development in pediatric patients with IBD. Growth failure occurs in 75% of Crohn's disease pediatric patients, while ulcerative colitis causes growth failure in 25%.[36] The pediatric patient with IBD should be evaluated at least twice yearly by a physician knowledgeable in all the necessary components of a comprehensive exam for these patients. The exam should include detailed body and weight measurements and appropriate laboratory testing. The list below outlines the necessary components of a comprehensive bi-yearly nutritional evaluation of pediatric patients with IBD. An aggressive nutritional program should be instituted, including supplements (it may be necessary to use injectable methods in some patients), one that is similar to the approach outlined for the adult patient, with the doses adjusted as appropriate.

Parents with children with IBD need to know the components necessary to monitor their children. They need not understand what the significance or even what the test is, but rather make sure that their children are being properly evaluated.

Monitoring of the Pediatric Patient with IBD

> Type and duration of inflammatory bowel disease; frequency of relapses
>
> Severity and extent of ongoing symptoms
>
> Medication history
>
> Three-day diet diary
>
> Physical examination
>
> > Height, weight, arm circumference, triceps skinfold measurements
>
> Evidence of increased disease activity (e.g., loss of subcutaneous fat, muscle wasting, edema, pallor, skin rash, liver enlargement)
>
> Laboratory tests
>
> > CBC and differential, reticulocyte and platelet count, sed rate, urinalysis

Serum total proteins, albumin, globulin, and retinol binding protein

Serum electrolytes, calcium, phosphate, ferritin, folate, carotenes, tocopherol, and B_{12}

Leukocyte ascorbate, magnesium, and zinc

Creatinine height index, BUN:creatinine ratio

The CDAI is not as accurate in monitoring IBD in children as it is in adults. To overcome this shortcoming, Lloyd-Still and Green devised a clinical scoring system for IBD in children.[46] The scoring system is divided into five major divisions (the maximum score in parentheses): general activity (10), physical examination and clinical complications (30), nutrition (20), x-rays (15), and laboratory (25). An elevated score (i.e., scores in the 80s) represents good status, while scores in the 30s and 40s represent severe disease. Table 8.4 outlines the criteria that are used to determine the clinical score.

Final Comments

In some individuals, Crohn's disease and ulcerative colitis are life-threatening diseases, which at times require emergency treatment. A small percentage of patients who have severe disease may require occasional hospitalization. Any serious increase in disease activity requires immediate medical attention. This is particularly true for individuals with IBD experiencing a fever of 101 degrees Fahrenheit or higher; profuse, constant, loose, bloody stools; loss of appetite; and a distended abdomen.

Table 8.4 Clinical Score in Chronic Pediatric IBD

General activity
10 Normal school attendance
<3 bowel movements per day
5 Lacks endurance
3–5 bowel movements per day
Misses <4 weeks school/year

Physical examination and complications

Abdomen:	10 Normal
	5 Mass
	1 Distension, tenderness
Proctoscope:	10 Normal, no fissures
	5 Friability, 1 fissure
	1 Ulcers, bleeding, fistulas, multiple fissures
Arthritis:	5 Nil
	3 One joint/arthralgia
	1 Multiple joints
Skin/stomatitis/eyes:	5 Normal
	3 Mild stomatitis
	4 Erythema nodosum, pyoderma, severe canker sores (stomatitis), inflammation of the eyes (uveitis)
Height:	10 > 2 inches/year
	5 <optimal %
	1 No growth
X-rays:	15 Normal
	10 Ileitis, colitis from the rectum to the splenic flexure (the turn of the colon near the spleen)
	5 Total colon or ileocecal involvement
	1 Toxic megacolon or obstruction

Laboratory

Hematocrit:	5 >40
	3 25–35
	1 <25
Erythrocyte sedimentation rate	5 Normal
	3 20–40
	1 >40
White blood cell count	5 Normal
	3 <20,000
	1 >20,000
Albumin	10 Normal
	5 3.0 g/dl
	1 < 2.5 g/dl

Dietary and Lifestyle Recommendations

- **Key recommendation: Identify and control food allergies.**
- Consume a diet that focuses on whole, unprocessed foods (whole grains, legumes, vegetables, fruits, nuts, and seeds).
- Eliminate your intake of alcohol, caffeine, and sugar.
- Identify and control food allergies.
- Get regular exercise.
- Perform a relaxation exercise (deep breathing, meditation, prayer, visualization, etc.) for 10 to 15 minutes each day.
- Drink at least 48 ounces of water daily.

Supplement Protocol

- High potency multiple vitamin and mineral formula
- Vitamin C: 3,000 mg to 8,000 mg each day
- Vitamin E: 200 to 400 IU daily
- Zinc: 30 to 45 mg daily
- Flaxseed oil: One tablespoon daily
- Pancreatin (8-10X): 350 to 700 mg three times daily between meals

References

Chapter 1. The Digestive System—Function and Analysis

1. Rubinstein E, et al.: Antibacterial activity of the pancreatic fluid. Gastroenterol 88:927–32, 1985.
2. Ransberger K: Enzyme treatment of immune complex diseases. Arthritis Rheuma 8:16–9, 1986.
3. Barrie S: Comprehensive Digestive Stool Analysis. In: A Textbook of Natural Medicine. Pizzorno JE and Murray MT (eds.). Bastyr University Publications, 1986.
4. Walker ARP, Walker BF, and Walker AJ: Faecal pH, dietary fibre intake and proneness to colon cancer in four South African populations. Br J Cancer 53:489–95, 1986.
5. Lee MJ and Barrie S: Relationship between butyrate pH and microbial flora in stool samples. Presented at the 16th International Congress on Microbial Ecology and Disease (Blacksburg, VA, USA) Sep 27–29, 1991.
6. Latella G and Caprilli R: Metabolism of the large bowel mucosa in health and disease. Int J Colorectal Dis (Germany) 6:127–32, 1991.
7. Roediger WE: The starved colon-diminished mucosal nutrition, diminished absorption and colitis. Dis Col Rect 75:713, 1982.

8. Jeejeebhoy KN, Royall D, and Wolever TMS: Clinical significance of colonic fermentation. Am J Gastroent 85:1307–12, 1990.

Chapter 2. Indigestion

1. Graham DY, Smith JL, and Patterson DJ: Why do apparently healthy people use antacid tablets? Am J Gastroenterol 78:257–60, 1983.

2. Bolla KI, Briefel G, Spector D, et al.: Neurocognitive effects of aluminum. Arch Neurol 49:1021–6, 1992.

3. Flaten TP: Geographical associations between aluminum and drinking water and death rates with dementia (including Alzheimer's disease), Parkinson's disease and amyotrophic sclerosis in Norway. Environ Geochem Health 12:152–7, 1990.

4. Perl DP, Gajdusek DC, Garruto RM, et al.: Intraneuronal aluminum accumulation in amyotrophic lateral sclerosis and Parkinsonism-dementia of Guam. Science 217:1053–5, 1982.

5. Weberg R and Berstad A: Gastrointestinal absorption of aluminum from single doses of aluminum containing antacids in man. Eur J Clin Invest 16:428–32, 1986.

6. Weberg R, et al.: Mineral-metabolic side effects of low-dose antacids. Scand J Gastroenterol 20:741–6, 1985.

7. Taylor GA, et al.: Gastrointestinal absorption of aluminum in Alzheimer's disease: Response to aluminum citrate. Age Ageing 21:81–90, 1992.

8. Grossman M, Kirsner J, and Gillespie I: Basal and histalog-stimulated gastric secretion in control subjects and in patients with peptic ulcer or gastric cancer. Gastroenterol 45:15–26, 1963.

9. Recker R: Calcium absorption and achlorhydria. New Engl J Med 313:70–3, 1985.

10. Nicar MJ and Pak CYC: Calcium bioavailability from calcium carbonate and calcium citrate. J Clin Endocrinol Metabol 61:391–3, 1985.

11. Editorial: Citrate for calcium nephrolithiasis. Lancet i:955, 1986.

12. Cushner HM, Copley JB, and Foulks CJ: Calcium citrate, a new phosphate-binding and alkalizing agent for patients with renal failure. Curr Ther Res 40:998–1004, 1986.

13. Barrie SA: Heidelberg pH capsule gastric analysis. In: Pizzorno JE and Murray MT: A Textbook of Natural Medicine. JBC Publications, Seattle, WA 1985.

14. Bray GW: The hypochlorhydria of asthma in childhood. Br Med. J I:181–97, 1930.

15. Rabinowitch IM: Achlorhydria and its clinical significance in diabetes mellitus. Am J Dig Dis 18:322-33, 1949.

16. Carper WM, Butler TJ, Kilby JO, and Gibson MJ: Gallstones, gastric secretion and flatulent dyspepsia. Lancet i:413–5, 1967.

17. Rawls WB and Ancona VC: Chronic urticaria associated with hypochlorhydria or achlorhydria. Rev Gastroent Oct:267–71, 1950.

18. Gianella RA, Broitman SA, and Zamcheck N: Influence of gastric acidity on bacterial and parasitic enteric infections. Ann Int Med 78:271–6, 1973.

19. De Witte TJ, Geerdink PJ, and Lamers CB: Hypochlorhydria and hypergastrinaemia in rheumatoid arthritis. Ann Rheum Dis 38:14–17, 1979.

20. Ryle JA and Barber HW: Gastric analysis in acne rosacea. Lancet ii:1195–6, 1920.

21. Ayres S: Gastric secretion in psoriasis, eczema and dermatitis herpetiformis. Arch Derm Jul:854–9, 1929.

22. Dotevall G and Walan A: Gastric secretion of acid and intrinsic factor in patients with hyper- and hypothyroidism. Acta Med Scand 186:529–33, 1969.

23. Howitz J and Schwartz M: Vitiligo, achlorhydria, and pernicious anemia. Lancet i:1331–4, 1971.

24. Howden CV and Hunt RH: Relationship between gastric secretion and infection. Gut 28:96–107, 1987.

25. Rafsky HA and Weingarten M: A study of the gastric secretory response in the aged. Gastroenterol May:348–52, 1946.

26. Davies D and James TG: An investigation into the gastric secretion of a hundred normal persons over the age of sixty. Br J Med i:1–14, 1930.

27. Baron JH: Studies of basal and peak acid output with an augmented histamine meal. Gut 3:136–44, 1963.

28. Mojaverian P, et al.: Estimation of gastric residence time of the Heidelberg capsule in humans. Gastroenterol 89:392–7, 1985.

29. Wright J: A proposal for standardized challenge testing of gastric acid secretory capacity using the Heidelberg capsule

180   *Stomach Ailments and Digestive Disturbances*

1979.

30. Berstad K and Berstad A: *Helicobacter pylori* infection in peptic ulcer disease. Scand J Gastroenterol 28:561-7, 1993.

31. Sarker SA and Gyr K: Non-immunological defense mechanisms of the gut. Gut 33:987-93, 1992.

32. Stockbruegger RW, et al.: Intragastric nitrites, nitrosamines, and bacterial overgrowth during cimetidine therapy. Gut 23:1048-54, 1982.

33. Shibata T, et al.: High acid output may protect the gastric mucosa from injury caused by *Helicobacter pylori* in duodenal ulcer patients. J Gastroenterol Hepatol 11:674-80, 1996.

34. Rokkas T, et al.: *Helicobacter pylori* infection and gastric juice vitamin C levels. Digestive Dis Sci 40:615-21, 1995.

35. Phull PS, et al.: Vitamin E concentrations in the human stomach and duodenum—correlation with *Helicobacter pylori* infection. Gut 39:31-5, 1996.

36. Baik SC, et al.: Increased oxidative DNA damage in *Helicobacter pylori*-infected human gastric mucosa. Cancer Res 56:1279-82, 1996.

37. van Marle J, et al.: Deglycyrrhizinised liquorice (DGL) and the renewal of rat stomach epithelium. Eur J Pharmacol 72:219-25, 1981.

38. Johnson B and McIssac R. Effect of some anti-ulcer agents on mucosal blood flow. Br J Pharmacol 1:308, 1981.

39. Kassir ZA: Endoscopic controlled trial of four drug regimens in the treatment of chronic duodenal ulceration. Irish Med J 78:153-6, 1985.

40. Morgan AG, et al.: Maintenance therapy: A two year comparison between Caved-S and cimetidine treatment in the prevention of symptomatic gastric ulcer. Gut 26:599-602, 1985.

41. Morgan AG, et al.: Comparison between cimetidine and Caved-S in the treatment of gastric ulceration, and subsequent maintenance therapy. Gut 23:545-51, 1982.

42. Glick L: Deglycrrhizinated liquorice in peptic ulcer. Lancet ii:817, 1982.

43. Beil W, Birkholz C, and Sewing KF: Effects of flavonoids on parietal cell acid secretion, gastric mucosal prostaglandin production and *Helicobacter pylori* growth. Arzneim Forsch 45:697-700, 1995.

44. Feldman H and Gilat T: A trial of deglycyrrhizinated liquorice in the treatment of duodenal ulcer. Gut 12:499–51, 1971.
45. Kang JY, et al.: Effect of colloidal bismuth subcitrate on symptoms and gastric histology in non-ulcer dyspepsia: A double-blind placebo-controlled study. Gut 31:476–80, 1990.
46. Marshall BJ, et al.: Bismuth subsalicylate suppression of *Helicobacteria pylori* in non-ulcer dyspepsia: A double-blind placebo-controlled trial. Dig Dis Scie 38:1674–80, 1993.
47. Oelgoetz AW, et al.: The treatment of food allergy and indigestion of pancreatic origin with pancreatic enzymes. Am J Dig Dis Nutr 2:422–6, 1935.

Chapter 3. Peptic Ulcers

1. Ateshkadi A, Lam NP, and Johnson CA: *Helicobacter pylori* and peptic ulcer disease. Clin Pharm 12:34–48, 1993.
2. Rydning A, et al.: Prophylactic effects of dietary fiber in duodenal ulcer disease. Lancet 2:736–9, 1982.
3. Kang JY, et al.: Dietary supplementation with pectin in the maintenance treatment of duodenal ulcer. Scand J Gastroenterol 23:95–9, 1988.
4. Harju E and Larme TK: Effect of guar gum added to the diet of patients with duodenal ulcers. J Parenteral Enteral Nutr 9:496–500, 1985.
5. Andre C, et al.: Evidence for anaphylactic reactions in peptic ulcer and varioliform gastritis. Ann Allergy 51:325–8, 1983.
6. Siegel J: Immunologic approach to the treatment and prevention of gastrointestinal ulcers. Ann Allergy 38:27–9, 1977.
7. Kumar N, et al.: Effect of milk on patients with duodenal ulcers. Br Med J 293:666, 1986.
8. Werbach MR: Nutritional Influences on Illness. Third Line Press, Tarzana, CA, 1987.
9. Cheney G: Rapid healing of peptic ulcers in patients receiving fresh cabbage juice. Cal Med 70:10–14, 1949.
10. Cheney G: Anti-peptic ulcer dietary factor. J Am Diet Assoc 26:668–72, 1950.
11. Glick L: Deglycrrhizinated liquorice in peptic ulcer. Lancet ii:817, 1982.

12. Tewari SN and Wilson AK: Deglycyrrhizinated liquorice in duodenal ulcer. Practitioner 210:820–5, 1972.
13. Morgan AG, et al.: Comparison between cimetidine and Caved-S in the treatment of gastric ulceration, and subsequent maintenance therapy. Gut 23:545–51, 1982.
14. Kassir ZA: Endoscopic controlled trial of four drug regimens in the treatment of chronic duodenal ulceration. Irish Med J 78:153–6, 1985.
15. Turpie AG, Runcie J, and Thomson TJ: Clinical trial of deglycyrrhizinate liquorice in gastric ulcer. Gut 10:299–303, 1969.
16. Rees WDW, et al.: Effect of deglycyrrhizinated liquorice on gastric mucosal damage by aspirin. Scand J Gastroent 14:605–7, 1979.

Chapter 4. Small Intestine Disturbances

1. Auricchio S: Gluten-sensitive enteropathy and infant nutrition. J Ped Gastroenterol Nutr 2(Suppl 1):S304–9, 1983.
2. Auricchio S, et al.: Does breast feeding protect against the development of clinical symptoms of celiac disease in children? J Ped Gatroenterol Nutr 2:428–33, 1983.
3. Cole SG and Kagnoff MF: Celiac disease. Ann Rev Nutr 5:241–66, 1985.
4. Fallstrom SP, Winberg J, and Anderson HJ: Cow's milk malabsorption as a precursor of gluten intolerance. Acta Paediatrica Scand 54:101–15, 1965.
5. McNicholl B, et al.: History, genetics, and natural history of celiac disease—gluten enteropathy. In: Food, Nutrition and Evolution. Walker DN and Kretchmer N (eds). Masson, New York, 1981, pp 169–78.
6. Simons FJ: Celiac disease as a geographic problem. In: Food, Nutrition and Evolution. Walker DN and Kretchmer N (eds). Masson, New York, 1981, pp 179–200.
7. Love AHG, et al.: Zinc deficiency and celiac disease. In: Perspectives in Celiac Disease. McNicholl B, McCarthy CF, and Fotrell PF (eds). University Press, Baltimore, MD, 1978, pp 335–42.
8. Messer M, Anderson CM, and Hubbard L: Studies on the mechanism of destruction of the toxic action of wheat gluten in coeliac disease by crude papain. Gut 5:295–303, 1964.

9. Messer M and Baume PE: Oral papain in gluten intolerance. Lancet ii:1022, 1976.

10. Carroccio A, et al.: Pancreatic enzyme therapy in childhood celiac disease. A double-blind prospective randomized study. Dig Dis Sci 40:2555–2560, 1995.

11. Sawada Y, et al.: Polyamines in the intestinal lumen of patients with small bowel bacterial overgrowth. Biochem Soc Trans 22:392(S), 1994.

12. Henriksson AEK, et al.: Small intestinal bacterial overgrowth in patients with rheumatoid arthritis. Ann Rheum Dis 52:503–10, 1993.

13. Sarker SA and Gyr R: Non-immunological defense mechanisms of the gut. Gut 33:1331–7, 1990.

14. Saltzman JR, et al.: Bacterial overgrowth without clinical malabsorption in elderly hypochlorhydric subjects. Gastroenterol 106:615–23, 1994.

15. Rubinstein E, et al.: Antibacterial activity of the pancreatic fluid. Gastroenterol 88:927–32, 1985.

16. Husebye E: Gastrointestinal motility disorders and bacterial overgrowth. J Intern Med 237:419–27, 1995.

17. Russo A, Fraser R, and Horowitz M: The effect of acute hyperglycemia on small intestinal motility in normal subjects. Diabetologia 39:984–9, 1996.

18. Watanabe A, Obata T, and Nagashima H: Berberine therapy of hypertyraminemia in patients with liver cirrhosis. Acta Med Okayama 36:277–81, 1982.

19. Abe F, Nagata S, and Hotchi M: Experimental candidiasis in liver injury. Mycopathologia 100:37–42, 1987.

20. Cazzola P, Mazzanti P, and Bossi G: In vivo modulating effect of a calf thymus acid lysate on human T lymphocyte subsets and CD4+/CD8+ ratio in the course of different diseases. Curr Ther Res 42:1011–7, 1987.

21. Kouttab NM, Prada M, and Cazzola P: Thymomodulin: Biological properties and clinical applications. Medical Oncology and Tumor Pharmacotherapy 6:5–9, 1989.

22. Adetumbi MA and Lau BH: *Allium sativum* (garlic)—A natural antibiotic. Med Hypothesis 12:227–37, 1983.

23. Prasad G and Sharma VD: Efficacy of garlic (*Allium sativum*) treatment against experimental candidiasis in chicks. Br Vet J 136:448–51, 1980.

24. Neuhauser I and Gustus EL: Successful treatment of intestinal moniliasis with fatty acid resin complex. Arch Intern Med 93:53–60, 1954.
25. Stiles JC, et al.: The inhibition of *Candida albicans* by oregano. J Applied Nutr 47:96–102, 1995.
26. Collins EB and Hardt P: Inhibition of *Candida albicans* by *Lactobacillus acidophilus.* J Dairy Sci 63:830–2, 1980.
27. Bjarnason I, MacPherson A, and Hollander D: Intestinal permeability: An overview. Gastroenterol 108:1566–81, 1995.
28. Bjarnason I: Intestinal permeability. Gut 35:S18–22, 1994.
29. Madara JL, et al.: Structure and function of the intestinal epithelial barrier in health and disease. Monogr Pathol 31:306–24, 1990.
30. Rooney PJ, Jenkins RT, and Buchanan WW: A short review of the relationship between intestinal permeability and inflammatory bowel disease. Clin Exp Rheumatol 8:75–83, 1990.
31. Levine JB and Lukawski-Trubish D: Extraintestinal considerations in inflammatory bowel disease. Gastroenterol Clin North Am 24:633–46, 1995.

Chapter 5. Colon Disorders

1. Sonnenberg A and Koch TR: Epidemiology of constipation in the United States. Dis Colon Rectum 32:1–8, 1989.
2. Wijayanegara H, et al.: A clinical trial of hydroxyethylrutosides in the treatment of haemorrhoids of pregnancy. J Int Med Res 20:54–60, 1992.
3. Annoni F, et al.: Treatment of acute symptoms of haemorrhoidal disease with high dose O-(beta-hydroxyethyl)-rutoside. Minerva Medica 77:1663–8, 1986.
4. Saggloro A, et al.: Treatment of hemorrhoidal syndrome with mesoglycan. Min Diet Gastr 31:311–5, 1985.
5. Fernandez-Banares F, et al.: Sugar malabsorption in functional bowel disease: Clinical implications. Am J Gastroenterol 88:2044–50, 1993.
6. Jones V, et al.: Food intolerance: A major factor in the pathogenesis of irritable bowel syndrome. Lancet ii:1115–8, 1982.
7. Petitpierre M, Gumowski P, and Girard J: Irritable bowel syndrome and hypersensitivity to food. Annals Allergy 54:538–40, 1985.

8. Somerville K, Richmond C, and Bell G: Delayed release peppermint oil capsules (Colpermin) for the spastic colon syndrome: A pharmacokinetic study. Br J Clin Pharmacol 18:638–40, 1984.

9. Rees W, Evans B, and Rhodes J: Treating irritable bowel syndrome with peppermint oil. Br Med J ii:835–6, 1979.

10. Svedlund J, et al.: Upper gastrointestinal and mental symptoms in the irritable bowel syndrome. Scand J Gastroenterol 20:595–601, 1985.

11. Goldsmith G and Patterson M: Irritable bowel syndrome: Treatment update. Am Fam Phys 31:191–5, 1985.

12. Ryan W, Kelly M, and Fielding J: The normal personality profile of irritable bowel syndrome patients. Irish J Med Sci 153:127–9, 1984.

13. Narducci F, et al.: Increased colonic motility during exposure to a stressful situation. Dig Dis Sci 30:40–4, 1985.

14. Position paper, Health and Public Policy Committee, American College of Physicians: Biofeedback for gastrointestinal disorders. Ann Int Med 103:291–3, 1985.

15. Svedlund J, et al.; Controlled study of psychotherapy in irritable bowel syndrome. Lancet ii:589–92, 1983.

16. Hentges DJ (ed): Human Intestinal Microflora. In: Health and Disease. Academic Press, New York, 1983.

17. Metchnikoff E: The Prolongation of Life. Arna Press, New York, 1908 (1977 reprint).

18. Shahani KM and Ayebo AD: Role of dietary lactobacilli in gastrointestinal microecology. Am J Clin Nutr 33:2448–57, 1980.

19. Shahani KM and Friend BA: Nutritional and therapeutic aspects of lactobacilli. J Appl Nutr 36:125–52, 1984.

20. Perdigon G, et al.: Symposium: Probiotic bacteria for humans: Clinical systems for evaluation of effectiveness. Immune system stimulation by probiotics. J Dairy Sci 78:1597–1606, 1995.

21. Clements ML, et al.: Lactobacillus prophylaxis for diarrhea due to enterotoxinogenic *Escherichia coli*. Antimicrob Agents Chemotherap 20:104–8, 1981.

22. Dios Pozo-Olano JD, et al.: Effect of a lactobacilli preparation on traveler's diarrhea: A randomized, double blind clinical trial. Gastroenterol 74:829–30, 1978.

23. Thompson GE: Control of intestinal flora in animals and humans: Implications for toxicology and health. J Environ Path Toxicol 1:113–23, 1977.

24. Clements ML, Levine MM, and Ristaino PA: Exogenous lacto-bacilli fed to man: Their fate and ability to prevent diarrheal disease. Prog Food Nutr Sci 7:29–37, 1983.

25. Zoppi G, et al.: Oral bacteriotherapy in clinical practice: I. The use of different preparations in infants treated with antibiotics. Eur J Ped 139:18–21, 1982.

26. Gotz VP, et al.: Prophylaxis against ampicillin-induced diarrhea with a lactobacillus preparation. Am J Hosp Pharm 36:754–7, 1979.

27. Zoppi G, et al.: Oral bacteriotherapy in clinical practice: I. The use of different preparations in the treatment of acute diarrhea. Eur J Ped 139:22–4, 1982.

28. Hughes VL and Hillier SL: Microbiologic characteristics of lactobacillus products used for colonization of the vagina. Obstet Gynecol 75:244–8, 1990.

29. Tomomatsu H: Health effects of oligosaccharides. Food Technology October:61–5, 1994.

30. Gibson GR, et al.: Selective stimulation of bifidobacteria in the human colon by oligofructose and inulin. Gastroenterol 108:975–82, 1995.

31. Duke JA: Handbook of Medicinal Herbs. CRC Press, Boca Raton, FL 1985, pp 78, 238–9, 287–8.

32. Leung AY: Encyclopedia of Common Natural Ingredients Used in Food, Drugs, and Cosmetics. John Wiley & Sons, New York, 1980, pp 52–3, 189–90.

33. Chang HM and But PPH: Pharmacology and Applications of Chinese Materia Medica, Volume 2. World Scientific, Teaneck, NJ, 1987, pp 1029–40.

34. Hahn FE and Ciak J: Berberine. Antibiotics 3:577–88, 1976.

35. Amin AH, Subbaiah TV, and Abbasi KM: Berberine sulfate: Antimicrobial activity, bioassay, and mode of action. Can J Microbiol 15:1067–76, 1969.

36. Johnson CC, Johnson G, and Poe CF: Toxicity of alkaloids to certain bacteria. Acta Pharmacol Toxicol 8:71–8, 1952.

37. Kaneda Y, et al.: In vitro effects of berberine sulfate on the growth of *Entamoeba histolytica, Giardia lamblia,* and *Tricomonas vaginalis.* Ann Trop Med Parasitol 85:417–25, 1991.

38. Subbaiah TV and Amin AH: Effect of berberine sulfate on *Entamoeba histolytica.* Nature 215:527–8, 1967.

39. Ghosh AK: Effect of berberine chloride on *Leishmania donovani.* Ind J Med Res 78:407–16, 1983.

40. Majahan VM, Sharma A, and Rattan A: Antimycotic activity of berberine sulphate: An alkaloid from an Indian medicinal herb. Sabouraudia 20:79–81, 1982.

41. Sun D, Courtney HS, and Beachey EH: Berberine sulfate blocks adherence of Streptococcus pyogenes to epithelial cells, fibronectin, and hexadecane. Antimicrobial Agents Chemother 32:1370–4, 1988.

42. Sabir M and Bhide N: Study of some pharmacologic actions of berberine. Ind J Physiol Pharm 15:111–32, 1971.

43. Kumazawa Y, et al.: Activation of peritoneal macrophages by berberine alkaloids in terms of induction of cytostatic activity. Int J Immunopharmacol 6:587–92, 1984.

44. Gupta S: Use of berberine in the treatment of giardiasis. Am J Dis Child 129:866, 1975.

45. Bhakat MP, et al.: Therapeutic trial of berberine sulphate in non-specific gastroenteritis. Ind Med J 68:19–23, 1974.

46. Kamat SA: Clinical trial with berberine hydrochloride for the control of diarrhoea in acute gastroenteritis. J Assoc Physicians India 15:525–9, 1967.

47. Desai AB, Shah KM, and Shah DM: Berberine in the treatment of diarrhoea. Ind Pediatr 8:462–5, 1971.

48. Sharma R, Joshi CK, and Goyal RK: Berberine tannate in acute diarrhea. Ind Pediatr 7:496–501, 1970.

49. Choudry VP, Sabir M, and Bhide VN: Berberine in giardiasis. Ind Pediatr 9:143–6, 1972.

50. Kamat SA: Clinical trial with berberine hydrochloride for the control of diarrhoea in acute gastroenteritis. J Assoc Physicians India 15:525–9, 1967.

51. Gupta S: Use of berberine in treatment of giardiasis. Am J Dis Child 129:866, 1975.

52. Sack RB and Froehlich JL: Berberine inhibits intestinal secretory response of vibrio cholerae toxins and *Escherichia coli* enterotoxins. Infect Immun 35:471–5, 1982.

53. Khin-Maung-U, et al.: Clinical trial of berberine in acute watery diarrhoea. Br Med J 291:1601–5, 1985.

54. Rabbani GH, et al.: Randomized controlled trial of berberine sulfate therapy for diarrhea due to enterotoxigenic *Escherichia coli* and *Vibrio cholerae.* J Infect Dis 155:979–84, 1987.

55. Akhter MH, Sabir M, and Bhide NK: Possible mechanism of antidiarrhoeal effect of berberine. Ind J Med Res 70:233–41, 1979.

56. Tai YH, Feser JF, Mernane WG, and Desjeux JF: Antisecretory effects of berberine in rat ileum. Am J Physiol 241:G253–8, 1981.
57. Hladon B: Toxicity of berberine sulfate. Acta Pol Pharm 32:113–20, 1075.

Chapter 6. Food Allergies

1. Adams F: The Genuine Works of Hippocrates. Williams & Williams, Baltimore, 1939.
2. Wright JV: Healing with Nutrition. Rodale, Emmaus, PA, 1984.
3. Dickey LD: Clinical Ecology. Thomas, Springfield, MA, 1974.
4. Taub EL: Food Allergy and the Allergic Patient. Thomas, Springfield, MA, 1978.
5. Brostoff J and Challacombe SJ (eds.): Food Allergy and Intolerance. WB Saunders, Philadelphia, 1987.
6. McGovern JJ: Correlation of clinical food allergy symptoms with serial pharmacological and immunological changes in the patient's plasma. Ann Allergy 44:57, 1980.
7. Ader R (ed): Psychoimmunology. Academic Press, New York, 1981.
8. Dockhorn RJ and Smith TC: Use of a chemically defined hypoallergenic diet in the management of patients with suspected food allergy. Ann Allergy 47:264–66, 1981.
9. Rowe AH and Rowe A: Food Allergy: Its manifestations and control and the elimination diets. CC Thomas, Springfield, IL, 1972.
10. Metcalfe D: Food hypersensitivity. J All Clin Imm 73:749–61, 1984.
11. Coca AF: Art of investigating pulse diet record in familial nonreagenic food allergy. Ann Allergy 2:1, 1944.
12. Rinkel HJ, Randolph T, and Zeller M: Food Allergy. CC Thomas, Springfield, IL, 1951.
13. Rinkel RJ: Food Allergy IV. The function and clinical application of the rotary diversified diet. J Pediat 32:266, 1948.

Chapter 7. Dietary Guidelines

1. Howell E: Enzyme Nutrition. Avery Publishing, Wayne, NJ, 1985.
2. Mowrey D and Clayson D: Motion sickness, ginger, and psychophysics. Lancet i:655–7, 1982.

3. Grontved A and Hentzer E: Vertigo-reducing effect of ginger root. ORL 48:282–6, 1986.

4. Grontved A, et al.: Ginger root against seasickness. A controlled trial on the open sea. Acta Otolaryngol 105:45–9, 1988.

5. Fischer-Rasmussen W, et al.: Ginger treatment of hyperemesis gravidarum. Eur J Ob Gyn Reproductive Biol 38:19–24, 1990.

6. National Research Council: Diet and Health: Implications for Reducing Chronic Disease Risk. National Academy Press, Washington, D.C., 1989.

7. Mensink RP and Katan MB: Effect of dietary trans fatty acids on high-density and low-density lipoprotein cholesterol levels in health subjects. New Engl J Med 323:439–45, 1990.

8. Jostaba JN, et al.: Early exposure to cow's milk and solid foods in infancy, genetic predisposition, and risk of IDDM. Diabetes 42:288–95, 1993.

9. Beynen AC, Van der Meer R, and West CE: Mechanism of casein-induced hypercholesterolemia: Primary and secondary features. Atherosclerosis 60:291–3, 1986.

10. Carrol KK: Review of clinical studies on cholesterol-lowering response to soy protein. J Am Dietetic Assoc 91:820–7, 1991.

11. Schauss A: Dietary Fish Oil Consumption and Fish Oil Supplementation. In: A Textbook of Natural Medicine. Pizzorno JE and Murray MT (eds). Bastyr College Publications, Seattle, WA, 1991, pp V; fish oils: 1–7.

12. Stanto JL and Keast DR: Serum cholesterol, fat intake, and breakfast consumption in the United States adult population. J Am Coll Nutr 8:567–72, 1989.

Chapter 8. Inflammatory Bowel Disease

1. Levi AJ: Diet in the management of Crohn's disease. Gut 26:985–8, 1985.

2. Jarnerot J, Jarnmark I, and Nilsson K: Consumption of refined sugar by patients with Crohn's disease, ulcerative colitis, or irritable bowel syndrome. Scand J Gastroenterol 18:999–1002, 1983.

3. Mayberry JF, Rhodes J, and Newcombe RG: Increased sugar consumption in Crohn's disease. Digestion 20:323–6, 1980.

 4. Grimes DS: Refined carbohydrate, smooth-muscle spasm and diseases of the colon. Lancet i:395–7, 1976.

 5. Thornton JR, Emmett PM, and Heaton KW: Diet and Crohn's disease: Characteristics of the pre-illness diet. Br Med J 279:762–4, 1979.

 6. Heaton KW, Tornton JR, and Emmett PM: Treatment of Crohn's disease with an unrefined-carbohydrate, fiber-rich diet. Br Med J 279:764–6, 1979.

 7. Morain CO, Segal AW, and Levi AJ: Elemental diet as primary treatment of acute Crohn's disease: A controlled trial. Br Med J 288:1859–62, 1984.

 8. Harries AD, Danis V, Heatley RV, et al.: Controlled trial of supplemented oral nutrition in Crohn's disease. Lancet i:887–90, 1983.

 9. Axelsson C and Jarnum S: Assessment of the therapeutic value of an elemental diet in chronic inflammatory bowel disease. Scand J Gastroenterol 12:89–95, 1977.

10. Voitk AJ, Echave V, Feller JH, et al.: Experience with elemental diet in the treatment of inflammatory bowel disease. Arch Surg 107:329–33, 1973.

11. Workman EM, Jonmes A, Wilson AJ, and Hunter JO: Diet in the management of Crohn's disease. Human Nutr 38A:469–73, 1984.

12. Jones VA, Workman E, Freeman AH, et al.: Crohn's disease: maintenance of remission by diet. Lancet ii:177–80, 1985.

13. Rowe A and Uyeyama K: Regional enteritis—Its allergic aspects. Gastroenterol 23:554–71, 1953.

14. James AH: Breakfast and Crohn's disease. Br Med J 276:943–5, 1977.

15. Thornton JR, Emmett PM, and Heaton KW: Diet and ulcerative colitis. Br Med J 280:293–4, 1980.

16. Meyers S and Janowitz HD: Natural History of Crohn's disease: An analytical review of the placebo lesson. Gastroenterol 87:1189–92, 1984.

17. Mekhjian HS, et al.: Clinical features and natural history of Crohn's disease. Gastroenterol 77:898–906, 1979.

18. Malchow H, et al.: European cooperative Crohn's disease study (ECCDS): Results of drug treatment. Gastroenterol 86:249–66, 1984.

19. Donowitz M: Arachidonic acid metabolites and their role in inflammatory bowel disease. Gastroenterol 88:580–7, 1985.

20. Ford-Hutchinson AW: Leukotrienes: Their formation and role as inflammatory mediators. Fed Proc 44:25–9, 1985.

21. Sharon P and Stenson WF: Enhanced synthesis of leukotriene B4 by colonic mucosa in inflammatory bowel disease. Gastroenterol 86:453–60, 1984.

22. Musch MW, Miller RJ, Field M, and Siegel MI: Stimulation of colonic secretion by lipoxygenase metabolites of arachidonic acid. Science 217:1255–6, 1982.

23. Podolsky DK and Isselbacher KJ: Glycoprotein composition of colonic mucosa. Gastroenterol 87:991–8, 1984.

24. Kim YS and Byrd JC: Ulcerative colitis: A specific mucin defect? Gastroenterol 87:1193–5, 1984.

25. Boland CR, Lance P, Levin B, et al.: Abnormal goblet cell glycoconjugates in rectal biopsies associated with an increased risk of neoplasia in patients with ulcerative colitis: Early results of a prospective study. Gut 25:1364–71, 1984.

26. Hentges DJ (ed): Human Intestinal Microflora. In: Health and Disease. Academic Press, New York, 1983.

27. Marcus R and Watt J: Seaweeds and ulcerative colitis in laboratory animals. Lancet ii:489–90, 1969.

28. Grasso P, et al.: Studies on carrageenan and large bowel ulceration in mammals. Food Cosmet Toxicol 11:555–64, 1973.

29. Motet NK: Editorial: On animal models for inflammatory bowel disease. Gastroenterol 62:1269–71, 1972.

30. Bentiz KR, Goldberg L, and Coulston F: Intestinal effect of carrageenans in the rhesus monkey. Food Cosmet Toxicol 11:565–75, 1973.

31. Bonfils S: Carrageenan and the human gut. Lancet ii:414, 1970.

32. Levine JB and Lukawski-Trubish D: Extraintestinal considerations in inflammatory bowel disease. Gastroenterol Clin North Am 24:633–46, 1995.

33. Murray MT: The Healing Power of Herbs. Prima, Rocklin, CA, 1995, pp 243–52.

34. Rosenberg IH, Bengoa JM, and Sitrin MD: Nutritional aspects of inflammatory bowel disease. Ann Rev Nutr 5:463–84, 1985.

35. Heatley HV: Review: Nutritional implications of inflammatory bowel disease. Scand J Gastroenterol 19:995–8, 1984.

36. Motil KJ and Grand RJ: Nutritional management of inflammatory bowel disease. Ped Clinics North Amer 32:447–69, 1985.

37. Salyers AA, Kurtitza AP, and McCarthy RE: Influence of dietary fiber on the intestinal environment. Proc Soc Exp Biol Med 180:415–21, 1985.

38. Fleming CR, et al.: Zinc nutrition in Crohn's disease. Dig Dis Sci 26:865–70, 1981.

39. Main ANH, Russell RI, Fell GS, et al.: Clinical experience of zinc supplementation during intravenous nutrition in Crohn's disease: Value of serum and urine zinc measurements. Gut 23:984–91, 1982.

40. Elsborg L and Larsen L: Folate deficiency in chronic inflammatory bowel diseases. Scand J Gastroenterol 14:1019–24, 1979.

41. Hellberg R, Hulten L, and Bjorn-Rasmussen E: The nutritional and haematological status before and after primary and subsequent resectional procedures for classical Crohn's disease and Crohn's colitis. Acta Chir Scand 148:453–60, 1982.

42. Franklin JL and Rosenberg IH: Impaired folic acid absorption in inflammatory bowel disease: Effects of salicylasosulfapyridine (azulfidine). Gastroenterol 64:517–25, 1973.

43. Carruthers LB: Chronic diarrhea treated with folic acid. Lancet i:849–50, 1946.

44. Filipsson S, Hulten L, and Lindstedt G: Malabsorption of fat and vitamin B12 before and after intestinal resection for Crohn's disease. Scand J Gastroenterol 13:529–36, 1978.

45. Best WR, et al.: Development of a Crohn's disease activity index. Gastroenterol 70:439–44, 1976.

46. Lloyd-Still J and Green OC: A clinical scoring system for chronic inflammatory bowel disease in children. Dig Dis Sci 24:620–4, 1979.

Index